Praise for **KETOFAST**

"As the science underlying ketosis and fasting progresses, you can always trust Dr. Joseph Mercola to be on the cutting edge! Follow this enjoyable read to do keto and fasting the right way, and avoid the common pitfalls, many of which will shock you."

— **Steven R. Gundry, M.D.**, *New York Times* best-selling author of The Plant Paradox series; Medical Director, The International Heart and Lung Institute

"Dr. Mercola has done it again. Tapping into the latest research on fasting and ketogenic diets, he has crafted an easy-to-understand, efficient, and highly effective program that can deliver life-changing results."

— **Mark Sisson**, author of the *New York Times* bestseller *The Keto Reset Diet* and founder of Primal Kitchen foods

"KetoFast provides a well-researched, practical approach to safely produce the metabolic flexibility needed to improve health and free a person from obesity, diabetes, and other disorders of metabolism."

— **Michael T. Murray, N.D.**, co-author of *The Encyclopedia of Natural Medicine*

"It's sobering to think that the simple timing and composition of our food could, if broadly adopted, change the course of millions of lives. KetoFast is a practical guide to reclaiming your metabolic health."

— **Travis Christofferson**, author of *Tripping over the Truth: How the Metabolic Theory of Cancer Is Overturning One of Medicine's Most Entrenched Paradigms*

KETOFAST

ALSO BY DR. JOSEPH MERCOLA

KetoFast Cookbook (with Pete Evans)*

*Superfuel**

*Fat for Fuel**

The Fat for Fuel Ketogenic Cookbook (with Pete Evans)*

Effortless Healing

The No-Grain Diet

Sweet Deception

Dark Deception

The Great Bird Flu Hoax

Freedom at Your Fingertips

Generation XL

Healthy Recipes for Your Nutritional Type

*Available from Hay House
Please visit:

Hay House USA: www.hayhouse.com®
Hay House Australia: www.hayhouse.com.au
Hay House UK: www.hayhouse.co.uk
Hay House India: www.hayhouse.co.in

***

KETOFAST

REJUVENATE YOUR HEALTH WITH A STEP-BY-STEP GUIDE TO TIMING YOUR KETOGENIC MEALS

DR. JOSEPH MERCOLA

HAY HOUSE, INC.
Carlsbad, California • New York City
London • Sydney • New Delhi

Published in the United States by: Hay House, Inc.: www.hayhouse.com®
Published in Australia by: Hay House Australia Pty. Ltd.: www.hayhouse.com.au
Published in the United Kingdom by: Hay House UK, Ltd.: www.hayhouse.co.uk
Published in India by: Hay House Publishers India: www.hayhouse.co.in

Cover design: The Book Designers • *Interior design:* Nick C. Welch
Illustrations on pages 93 and 94: John Wiley and Sons, *Obesity Journal,*
Stephen D. Anton, Mark Mattson, et al.
Indexer: Jay Kreider

Library of Congress has cataloged the earlier edition as follows:

Names: Mercola, Joseph, author.
Title: Ketofast : rejuvenate your health with a step-by-step guide to timing
    your ketogenic meals / Dr. Joseph Mercola.
Description: Carlsbad, California : Hay House, Inc., [2019] | Includes
    bibliographical references and index.
Identifiers: LCCN 2019000138 | ISBN 9781401956790 (hardcover : alk. paper)
Subjects: LCSH: Fasting--Health aspects. | Ketogenic diet.
Classification: LCC RM226.5 .M46 2019 | DDC 613.2/5--dc23 LC record available
at https://lccn.loc.gov/2019000138

Tradepaper: ISBN: 978-1-4019-5763-6
E-book ISBN: 978-1-4019-5680-6
Audiobook ISBN: 978-1-4019-5681-3

10 9 8 7 6 5 4 3 2
1st edition, April 2019
2nd edition, August 2021

Printed in the United States of America

To my Mom and Dad, whom I recently lost.

Thank you both for raising me. I wouldn't be where I am today without your love and support.

CONTENTS

INTRODUCTION

You may be reading this book because you have a severe health challenge, or like 40 percent of the population, are obese. If you fall into either of those categories, this book will provide a strategy that will help you regain your healthy weight, with the absolutely liberating experience of finally being free of cravings that sabotage your ability to choose healthy foods.

The weight that you lose on this program will be mostly visceral fat, the dangerous fat around your organs that is believed to be a driver of metabolic dysfunction, insulin resistance, and chronic inflammation. Losing this fat will help lower your blood pressure, improve your cholesterol patterns to healthy ratios, and lower your risk of heart disease and diabetes.

The United States is suffering from an onslaught of chronic degenerative illnesses, and insulin resistance in particular is playing a major role in the epidemics of obesity, heart disease, cancer, and diabetes as well as neurodegenerative diseases like Alzheimer's and Parkinson's disease.

Even conservative conventional medical experts estimate that half of the U.S. population has diabetes or prediabetes, and if we utilize more sensitive estimates, such as a 70-gram oral glucose challenge and measure insulin levels over four hours, then we have to consider a whopping 80 percent of Americans as insulin-resistant.

Insulin resistance is invariably accompanied by metabolic inflexibility, or the inability to burn fat as a primary fuel. This is in large part due to two factors: an over-reliance on carbs and processed foods, and the timing of one's meals. These issues are covered in detail in my previous best-selling book, *Fat for Fuel*.

The problem with using carbs as your primary fuel is that they cause your blood sugar levels to rise and fall, which contributes to food cravings and makes it hard for your brain to stay focused for long periods of time. When you're metabolically flexible and can burn fat for fuel, your brain has a consistent fuel source that it can rely on, allowing you to focus for longer periods of time. You also won't have brain fog. The increased mental clarity is one of the most remarkable benefits that many people experience with metabolic flexibility.

Your ability to become metabolically flexible will be a foundational element for resolving most chronic health challenges you have. Once you are able to start burning fat for fuel, your body will generate far less oxidative stress, therefore reducing chronic inflammation. This is due to the production of ketones, which are very powerful anti-inflammatory molecules that will lower inflammatory markers such as C-reactive protein and white blood cell levels. This will improve common conditions like arthritis, acne, and eczema. It will also radically improve your gut microbiome, which will decrease your risk of one of the most common surgeries in the U.S.—having your gallbladder removed.

Once you can burn fat for fuel, you will typically have more than enough energy and greater endurance; you will no longer hit that proverbial wall in your energy. You will also sleep more soundly and tend to have longer and more frequent periods of deep sleep, which will help you feel more relaxed and rested when you wake up.

Most importantly, this approach will help you abolish insulin resistance, which, as we've discussed, is one of the fundamental contributing factors to the epidemic of heart disease, Alzheimer's, cancer, and diabetes that affects more than 80 percent of the population, causing so much pain, suffering, and premature death.

CYCLICAL KETOGENESIS: CYCLING IN AND OUT OF KETOSIS

I am a fond proponent of only recommending health strategies that I have carefully researched and personally implemented. Like many people who discover nutritional ketosis, I initially believed that it was the ideal dietary approach, and should be used continuously. However, my body taught me that this is not the case for me, and I believe that is also true for most people.

Continuous nutritional ketosis is a short-term intervention that is used for a few weeks to a few months (sometimes longer for those who are metabolically damaged and/or obese). You only need to do continuous nutritional ketosis until your body learns to burn your fat for fuel and begins to make ketones. Once you start creating ketones in significant amounts (over 0.5 mmol/l in your blood), you have regained your metabolic flexibility and need to start cycling in higher amounts of carbs and protein.

There are a number of serious health challenges that will typically result if you continue to eat a low-carb, adequate-protein, and high-quality-fat diet after you've established metabolic flexibility. One of the most important is that you will deprive your gut microbiome of the food it requires in the form of nondigestible fibers from the healthy forms of carbs found in vegetables and fruits that should be a part of a regular diet.

Please avoid the mistake I, and many others, have made with nutritional ketosis. Most of us should not be on a continuous keto diet; instead, it should only be done intermittently. Once you become metabolically flexible and are able to create ketones, it is ideal to eat a ketogenic diet only a few times a week, so you can maintain your metabolic flexibility. If you revert back to your previous high-carb and high-protein diet continuously, you will eventually lose your metabolic flexibility and be back to square one.

TIMING OF YOUR FOOD

Aside from carefully adjusting your macronutrient composition to achieve nutritional ketosis, a strategy that is almost as important is the *timing* of your food. Ideally, you'll want to gradually compress your eating window to six to eight hours a day. This is known as intermittent fasting, or time-restricted eating.

Most people eat continuously throughout their day, from the moment they wake up until just before going to bed. Many have not taken a break from constant grazing for years or even decades. This violates our genetic and biochemical programming and deprives us of the many magnificent benefits that cycling in and out of eating provides.

Until the last hundred years or so, we have not had 24/7 access to food. (Of course, in some parts of the world, this is still the case). But modern technology has now made it possible for so many of us to eat food around the clock. The problem is that even the highest-quality, most nutrient-dense food will inhibit your ability to achieve optimal health if you eat without a break. You simply must regularly refrain from continuous eating if you are going to activate your body's innate repair and regeneration mechanisms.

If you are new to intermittent fasting, the first window of time to address is the period before you go to bed. It is crucial to stop eating food for at least three hours before you go to sleep, so that you aren't providing calories your body has no need for. If your body has access to calories it doesn't need to use right away, it will cause a backup in your production of adenosine triphosphate (ATP)—the energy currency of your body—in your mitochondria. This will result in the production of excess free radicals that can damage your cell membranes, proteins, and DNA.

BENEFITS OF KETOFASTING OR PARTIAL FASTING

Once you have started to reap the benefits of cyclical ketosis discussed above and are finally able to burn fat for fuel, you can take your program to the next level by integrating KetoFast or partial fasting.

You might be wondering why you would want to do that if you are already burning fat for fuel and regularly engaging in intermittent fasting with a compressed eating window. The primary reason is that intermittent fasting, even 18 hours a day, is not going to be enough to trigger the magical benefits achieved from going through longer periods without food.

There are three major benefits that you will reap by KetoFasting:

1. **Detoxification.** You will facilitate the removal of the toxins that we have all been exposed to over the past century. Most of these toxins are fat-soluble and stored in your fat cells. When you go through periods with limited foods and have metabolic flexibility (i.e., are capable of burning fat for fuel), you will start to burn your visceral fat stores, which are loaded with toxins, and liberate them so the toxins can be processed and eliminated.

2. **Stem Cell Activation.** Stem cells are cells from which all other cells with specialized functions are generated. They provide the raw material to replace damaged or diseased cells in your body, and when you engage in longer periods of fasting, you stimulate their production.

3. **Autophagy.** *Autophagy* literally means "self-eating"; it's your body's natural process of cleaning house. Autophagy removes damaged proteins and clears damaged cellular parts, such as mitochondria. It also plays a role in eliminating pathogens. Autophagy is a vital metabolic strategy for cellular repair and regeneration and important to maximize your health.

The KetoFast program will provide your body with the nutritional support and strategies you need to ensure that the toxins you release during the fast are properly metabolized. When you become metabolically flexible and are able to burn fat for fuel, you will engage in a process called lipolysis, which is the breaking down of fats. Once the fat is liberated from your cells, so are the toxins that were dissolved in that fat. This creates a potentially dangerous metabolic scenario for most people, as they simply do not have the nutrients to support the detoxification process, which occurs primarily in the liver and extends to the four organs of elimination: colon, skin, kidneys, and lungs. Supplying the necessary nutrients to the liver and providing specific support to the organs of elimination is an essential aspect of "scientific fasting." This is especially important in today's toxic world, where all of us are exposed to a wide range of toxic chemicals and hormones that didn't exist in previous generations.

The purpose of detoxification is to convert the fat-soluble toxins to water-soluble material that can ultimately be excreted in your sweat, urine, or stool. If your body is not supported in this process, the liberated toxins will wreak metabolic havoc in your body, and will likely be reabsorbed, causing you more problems in the future.

KETOFASTING VS. WATER FASTING

I used to believe that multiple-day water fasting was one of the most powerful metabolic interventions I had ever encountered. But after studying the process more carefully, I realized there were a few major problems with it.

The obvious one is compliance. I realized that unless someone was seriously ill, they would be unlikely to have the discipline required to implement such a rigorous intervention, and that compliance to the program would be limited at best. The beauty of KetoFasting is that compliance is not really an issue, as you gradually build up to the point where you are comfortable without eating for 16 to 18 hours. From there, it is a relatively easy transition to eat only one 300- to 600-calorie meal for another 24 hours. This is largely because your body has adapted to burning fat for fuel and you really don't have any hunger cravings.

The other benefit is that you can complete far more partial fast days in a year than you can multiday water fasts, so that all the benefits of fasting that are described in the section above will occur on a far more frequent basis.

You also get to look forward to eating more carbs and protein on the day following your partial fast! The extra protein and carbs will help you rebuild your body, which is exactly what you need and deserve. Most of the metabolic magic of fasting occurs during the refeeding phase after you have activated your stem cells and targeted damaged subcellular structures for removal with autophagy. This is similar to what happens in exercises like strength-training in which you intentionally damage your tissue and subsequently improve it when you allow your body adequate time to rest and recover.

Finally, one of the most important reasons to opt for Keto-Fasting rather than water fasting is that KetoFasting allows you to more carefully support your body's detoxification systems as they metabolize the fat-soluble toxins released during the fasting phase, so they can be properly eliminated from your body and not reabsorbed.

RESOURCES TO HELP YOU

I have written an accompanying recipe book, the *KetoFast Cookbook*, with the world-class Australian chef Pete Evans. The recipes are based on my specifications for your 300- to 600-calorie partial fast day.

The foods in the recipes are loaded with phytochemicals that will support your detoxification during the KetoFast, and should serve to eliminate virtually all the side effects that people experience with fasting.

YOU HAVE AN EXCITING JOURNEY IN FRONT OF YOU

I am beyond excited for you to implement what I consider to be one of the most powerful physical strategies to not only help you recover your health but also improve it to levels you likely never believed were possible. This will be an exciting journey for you, and I encourage you to solicit all the support you can from friends and family members. Invite them to join you on your journey so they too can reap all these magnificent improvements in health and avoid the pitfalls of relying on prescription drugs that never address the root cause of disease.

CHAPTER 1

WHY WE GET SICK

High-tech, drug-based Western medicine excels in surgical procedures, emergency interventions, sophisticated diagnosis, invasive procedures, and other such interventions. But when it comes to chronic health problems, modern medicine falls woefully short of providing effective help, and unfortunately, in many cases, prescribing drugs for chronic problems actually harms the patient. Are you tired of leaving just about every doctor visit with a prescription in hand? Or being told they can find nothing wrong with you, with the implication being that whatever is troubling you is in your head?

Or worse, perhaps you've been given a name for your condition but have then been told there's nothing the doctor can do to treat it—the old "diagnose and adios" approach to medicine. And now you're on your own, with a name for your condition but no tools to address it. Conventional medicine is fairly effective at diagnosing illnesses. Where it fails miserably is recommending treatments that address the foundational cause of the problem. When you walk away with only a prescription in hand, you're leaving your doctor's office without knowing how to get to the source of the problem to fix it for good. Instead, you're left to cover up the symptoms with pharmaceuticals—or worse, more invasive or toxic procedures—for the rest of your life.

At best, being given a diagnosis, then rushed out the door with one or several prescriptions is a lonely place to be. If you have cancer or another serious illness, it can feel like a death sentence.

Despite the feelings of isolation this experience can stir up, if you have been diagnosed with a chronic disease, you are not alone. According to the U.S. Centers for Disease Control and Prevention (CDC), *half* of all Americans suffer from at least one chronic illness.[1] That's nearly 164 million people in the U.S. alone. Even more concerning, chronic diseases have quadrupled among children since the 1960s.

So what does "chronic disease" include? All the top killers, for starters: cancer, cardiovascular disease, stroke, Alzheimer's, type 2 diabetes, and obesity. It also includes chronic conditions that can make life challenging and even a burden at times, like arthritis, Parkinson's, multiple sclerosis (MS), Lyme disease, fibromyalgia, chronic fatigue, dementia, and autism. Chronic disease is now the leading cause of death and disability in America. Cardiovascular and cerebrovascular diseases contribute to the greatest decline in quality of life after 65 and are directly responsible for about one-third of all deaths. In fact, *7 of the top 10 causes of death in 2014 were chronic diseases.* Cancer and heart disease alone accounted for nearly 46 percent of all deaths in that year.

Chronic disease also greatly contributes to the rising health-care costs in America, as 90 cents of every dollar spent on health care goes toward the treatment of someone with a chronic disease. From an economic standpoint, a 90 percent growth in Medicare spending can be attributed to chronic disease alone, with the total cost of chronic disease projected to reach $42 trillion by 2030.[2]

While the U.S. ranks number one by a huge margin in healthcare expenditures, it ranks *70th* in quality of health. *Clearly, our current methods aren't working!* Obviously, the traditional healthcare system fails to effectively address chronic disease. As more and more people develop chronic disease—even multiple chronic diseases—doctors are increasingly unable to provide solutions that actually work.

I sincerely believe most physicians truly intend to help their patients. However, the tools available to them in their conventional medicine tool chest simply don't include one of the most effective strategies for preventing, diagnosing, *and reversing* chronic disease—empowering your body to heal itself through periodic fasts.

But before I can explain exactly why fasting is such a powerful healing tool, it's crucial to understand just what's making us so sick in the first place. In many ways, that is what I have been doing for the past four decades. But in the past two years, my understanding has evolved and expanded to reveal that the key to reversing this devastating trend has been hiding in plain sight in the scientific literature. It's just that in this era of highly specialized science, few of us have the time to read all the relevant literature, let alone organize the information found within it in useful and critical ways. Through my intensive deep dives into recent studies, I have come to appreciate that it is helpful to look at the underlying molecular biological mechanisms that contribute to chronic disease in order to understand how to reduce, and yes, even reverse it.

To do that, you have to start by examining how the food you've been introducing into your body has evolved over the past several decades, and how this may have contributed to chronic disease. From there, you can develop a plan for how to rectify the damage these kinds of foods have caused and promote your body's innate ability to heal and stay in *homeostasis*—the scientific term for "balance"—without the need for prescriptions or other traditional medical interventions.

DIETARY CHANGES—COMPOSITION, QUALITY, AND TIMING

Since the beginning of the 20th century, the average American has steadily increased consumption of industrially processed fats (think vegetable oils, such as canola, soy, and corn oil). There are multiple problems with these relatively new kinds of fats. At the top of the list is that the primary type of fats they contain are omega-6.

To be clear, omega-6 oils are essential to your health. Along with omega-3 fats, they are a polyunsaturated fatty acid (PUFA). But omega-6 fats are typically proinflammatory and contribute to insulin resistance (which I will cover in just a moment). They can also alter your mood and impair learning and cell repair.

Because the omega-6 vegetable oils have been promoted as healthy by the media and the health establishment, and because they are used in so many processed foods, the typical American is eating far too many omega-6 fats compared to omega-3 fats. But you need an optimal *balance* of omega-3 to omega-6 fats if you want to achieve high levels of health. The ideal ratio of omega-3 to omega-6 fats ranges from 1:1 to 1:5, but the typical Western diet is staggeringly off-balance, at between 1:20 and 1:50.

Omega-6 fats are also chemically unstable and prone to oxidative damage. These damaged oils are then incorporated into your cell membranes, making your cells fragile and prone to oxidation.

Another fat-related diet development is that over the past several decades, saturated fat has been mistakenly labeled the enemy of good health, and Americans have been counseled to make whole grains the mainstay of their diet. The problem here is that grains are high in carbohydrates, and eating excess carbs generates a rapid rise in blood glucose. Because excess glucose is toxic to your cells, your pancreas will secrete insulin into your bloodstream in order to reduce blood glucose levels.

If you continue to eat a diet that it is high in sugar and grains, over time your insulin receptors become desensitized to insulin, requiring more and more insulin to get the job done. This is referred to as insulin resistance, and it is one of the most pervasive factors contributing to disease. According to Dr. Joseph Kraft in his book *Diabetes Epidemic & You*, about 80 percent of Americans now have it. This is significant because insulin resistance is a powerful precursor to many chronic diseases including cancer, heart disease, obesity, and type 2 diabetes. Insulin resistance also cues your liver to manufacture toxic fats known as ceramides, which can then cross the blood-brain barrier and cause oxidation, inflammation, and cell death in the brain.[3]

In addition to eating too many omega-6 fats and high-carb foods, most of us simply eat too much food, and too often. In fact, the vast majority of Americans eat *all day long*[4]—with as many as 15.5 separate eating events in a typical day. Most also consume a majority of their daily calories late in the evening, which is exactly when your body requires the *least* amount of energy as calories from food. That's why I recommend you avoid eating for at least three hours before bedtime—and that includes *everyone*, no matter what kind of diet you follow or don't follow, or whether you are a proponent of fasting or following a particular fasting regimen or not. A continuous consumption of food will prevent you from ever reaping the benefits of going without food.

Avoiding food for three hours before going to bed optimizes your mitochondrial function and helps prevent cellular damage. After all, sleep is when your body repairs itself and performs important detox functions. If it is forced to digest a meal while you sleep, it will forgo these vital processes. That's why I typically stop eating four to six hours before I go to bed, although a three-hour window is also beneficial, and probably more doable for most people.

SYNTHETIC FERTILIZERS

Another fairly recent change in dietary habits is the addition of chemical fertilizers. Developed in order to help farmers grow more crops, they have decimated the diversity of microbes in the soil and depleted minerals as well. This means that food produced with their help delivers fewer crucial nutrients, which, over time, contributes to deficiencies and imbalances within your body.

These fertilizers also enabled farmers to forgo the traditional method of crop rotation—a strategy that replaced soil nutrients—and grow only those crops that were in high demand and heavily subsidized, such as corn and soy. So, as our soil microbes became less diverse, so did our food supply. Once we had all that corn and soy, we had to find use for them, which is another reason why consumption of omega-6-heavy corn oil and soybean oil has skyrocketed over the past several decades.

FOOD ADDITIVES

These now-ubiquitous chemicals were first developed in the first half of the 20th century to extend shelf life and improve the flavor of foods that were becoming increasingly processed. Chemicals were added to the food supply at a record clip during that time. By 1958, there were 800 different chemicals in use. Today there are an estimated 10,000 chemicals commonly used in the food supply.

At least 1,000 of the current food additives have never been reviewed for safety by the Food and Drug Administration (FDA) thanks to a loophole known as "generally regarded as safe" (GRAS). This means that if an additive was in use before the FDA passed the Food Additives Amendment of 1958, it is perfectly legal to keep using it.[5] One type of food additive that has wreaked the most havoc is trans fat, which we now know is a prime driver of inflammation and linked to heart disease,[6] insulin resistance,[7] obesity,[8] and Alzheimer's disease.[9]

PESTICIDES, PARTICULARLY GLYPHOSATE

Glyphosate is the active ingredient in the pervasive herbicide Roundup. Its usage on crops to control weeds in the U.S. and elsewhere has increased dramatically in the past two decades. This increase was driven by the escalation of genetically modified (GM) crops in that same time period, the widespread emergence of glyphosate-resistant weeds among the GM crops (necessitating ever-higher doses to achieve the same herbicidal effect), as well as the increased adoption of glyphosate as a desiccating agent just before harvest.

Glyphosate is an enormous threat to your health. The increase in glyphosate usage in the U.S. is extremely well correlated with the concurrent increase in the incidence and/or death rate of multiple diseases, including thyroid cancer, liver cancer, bladder cancer, pancreatic cancer, kidney cancer, and myeloid leukemia. The World Health Organization (WHO) revised its assessment of glyphosate's carcinogenic potential in March 2015, relabeling it as a "probable carcinogen."[10, 11, 12, 13, 14]

This is dire news, given that nearly 2 million tons of glyphosate were dumped into American soil from 1974 to 2016,[15] and nearly 10 million tons were applied worldwide in that same time frame.

Glyphosate negatively impacts health in many ways:

- It disrupts delicate hormonal balance by binding with estrogen receptors.

- It is toxic to your gut microbes, which play such an important role in inflammation, immunity, digestion and mental health.

- And perhaps most perniciously, it impairs mitochondrial function and makes your mitochondria more prone to oxidative damage (I will dive further into mitochondrial health in just a moment).

ELECTROMAGNETIC FIELDS

You swim daily in a sea of electromagnetic fields (EMFs). You are exposed to EMFs all day long, not only in public, but also within your home. EMFs come from many sources, including cellphones, cell towers, computers, baby monitors, microwaves, smart appliances, Bluetooth devices, and Wi-Fi, to name just a few.

It's not just my opinion that EMFs are a public health menace; there is considerable science that documents the dangers that EMFs pose to human, animal, and environmental health. Up until very recently, I believed that living a healthy lifestyle and following a healthy diet, exercise, and supplement program would be more than enough to protect most people from EMF-related dangers. But I have come to realize that as powerful as optimizing your nutrition is, implementing dietary changes without also addressing your EMF exposure is the equivalent of putting fingers in holes on a sinking ship.

Few of us are more than two feet from our cellphones at any given time—even when we sleep. We spend most of our working hours within arm's reach of a computer that is wirelessly connected to the Internet. We live in homes, neighborhoods, and cities that are in direct and constant contact with EMFs via electrical wiring, microwave ovens, cellphone towers, and Wi-Fi. We have embraced these technologies and woven them into the fabric of our lives without much, if any, regard for the damage they can do physically and emotionally.

Very few people are seriously concerned about the negative health effects of EMF exposure, which include genetic mutations, cellular dysfunction, and disease. And our exposure is only continuing to grow. Consider how many people you see each day looking at their cellphones instead of looking at the faces of friends or family who are right beside them.

Martin Pall, Ph.D., professor emeritus of biochemistry and basic medical sciences at Washington State University, has identified and published several papers describing the speculated mechanisms of how EMFs from cellphones and wireless technologies damage humans, animals, and plants.[16] Research suggests intracellular calcium increases with exposure to EMFs. It is the excess calcium in the cell and increased calcium signaling that are responsible for generating excessive oxidative stress that causes unrepaired DNA damage.

When there's excess calcium in the cell, it increases levels of both nitric oxide (NO) and superoxide. While NO has many beneficial health effects, excessive amounts are dangerous as it reacts with superoxide, forming peroxynitrites, then damages cell membranes, DNA, mitochondria, and protein. These biologic insults contribute to accelerated aging and radically increase the risk of developing chronic disease.

The prevalence of EMFs provides all the more reason to eat as healthfully as possible in order to optimize your body's mechanisms of repair and regeneration! (And if you are wondering what you can do specifically about mitigating the damage of EMFs, know that I am currently at work on a book about how to protect yourself from them. You can also sign up for my newsletter at mercola.com, where I regularly share information on this topic.)

EXCESS IRON

Many believe that iron is a useful mineral to supplement. If you are a woman in your reproductive years, perhaps you have even been diagnosed with an iron deficiency at some point. The problem with iron is that other than through menstruation, your body has no way to purge excess amounts of it. With the near ubiquity of iron-fortified foods, and high red meat consumption (meat is a prominent source of iron), over time your iron levels can build up to toxic levels.

Excess iron impairs your health by acting as a catalyst that transforms hydrogen peroxide (which is produced as a by-product of cellular respiration) into hydroxyl radical—a dastardly free radical that decimates mitochondrial DNA, proteins, and membranes. It also contributes to increased inflammation throughout your body, which is a precursor to all manner of chronic diseases. The best way to reduce excess iron is to donate blood or have a therapeutic phlebotomy performed if you have conditions that don't allow you to donate blood.

MICROBIOME CHANGES

Recent estimates suggest your body houses some 30 trillion bacteria[17] and about 1 quadrillion viruses (bacteriophages). These microbes perform a wide variety of useful functions, including digestion, immunity, modulating inflammation, and promoting mental health (since the gut and brain are so connected). Devastatingly, many factors, including some I'm covering in this chapter, can harm microbiome health:

- High-carb diets can cause pathogenic bacteria, such as *H. pylori* and yeast, which feed on glucose, to increase dramatically, crowding out the beneficial bacteria that reside in your GI tract.

- Antibiotic use can kill off beneficial bacteria, resulting in an overgrowth of disease-causing species that are destructive to both gut and brain health.

- Gut-disrupting medications, such as commonly prescribed proton pump inhibitors, are also responsible for upsetting this delicate balance.

- The chlorine in unfiltered municipal tap water can impair your microbiome.

- Research is slowly building the case that artificial sweeteners can lower the number of beneficial bacteria.

INFLAMMATION

A diet high in carbohydrates, including sugars, fans the flames of inflammation in your body, as it produces 30 to 40 percent more reactive oxygen species (ROS) than when you follow an eating protocol that promotes burning fat for your primary fuel—as both fasting and following a high-fat (saturated fat, not omega-6 fats, which tend to be inflammatory), low-net-carb, moderate-protein diet (as I outlined in my book *Fat for Fuel*) promote. Research shows that low-carb diets tend to reduce levels of systemic inflammation.[18]

Impaired Mitochondrial Health

Mitochondria are the organelles within your cells that are responsible for converting the food you eat to forms of usable energy, such as adenosine triphosphate (ATP), which fuels all the many processes of your body. They do so by metabolizing the sugars and fats you eat, ultimately shuttling the electrons from the sugars and fats to oxygen, to form carbon dioxide and water. And they do it relentlessly—your mitochondria produce about 110 pounds of ATP *every day.*[19]

You simply can't have overall health without mitochondrial health. And all the factors I've listed in this chapter place your mitochondria under attack. The good news is that healing mitochondrial dysfunction offers one of the simplest and most promising new strategies for improving your health and helping prevent diseases like cancer from developing in your body in the first place.

The process your mitochondria use to produce ATP is called oxidative phosphorylation, and one of the by-products of these processes is reactive oxygen species (ROS). These unstable atoms have one or more unpaired electrons, and can form destructive free radicals. Free radicals seek to steal electrons from other molecules in an effort to stabilize themselves. This process can create an army of hungry free radicals that can then degrade the membranes, proteins, and DNA of your mitochondria.

Free radicals can also damage your DNA by disrupting replication, interfering with its maintenance activities, and altering its structure. Research estimates that your DNA suffers a free radical attack somewhere between 10,000 and 100,000 times a day, or nearly *one assault every second.*[20]

All of these factors can lead to tissue degradation, which increases your risk of disease. In fact, free radicals are linked to more than 60 different diseases, including heart disease, cancer, and neurodegenerative diseases like Alzheimer's and Parkinson's disease.

Surprisingly, free radicals also play a role in health—not just disease. In particular, they regulate many crucial cellular functions, such as the creation of melatonin and nitric oxide, and the optimization of important pathways that regulate functions such as hunger, fat storage, and aging.

TIMING

Dr. Satchin Panda, a leading researcher in circadian rhythm at the Salk Institute for Biological Studies in San Diego and author of *The Circadian Code: Lose Weight, Supercharge Your Energy, and Sleep Well Every Night*, has found that only about 10 percent of Americans eat all their food within a 12-hour window.[21] I was shocked when I heard this number, because it means that people are eating during nearly all of their waking hours. In fact, Dr. Panda's research found that Americans typically eat nearly 15 out of the 24 hours in a day, and that they consume more than 35 percent of their calories after 6 P.M., when energy needs are lowest. This type of nonstop eating kicks off a host of serious health consequences because we simply weren't designed to eat food at all hours of the day, especially in the three hours before you sleep.

> *Only about 10 percent of Americans eat all their food within a 12-hour window.*

Think of your ancient ancestors. They couldn't amble over to the fridge whenever they felt the faintest hunger pang, or were bored. Hunting, gathering, and growing food did not provide a reliable stream of calories. Even when food was plentiful, it typically took some serious time and effort to make it edible. As a result of the way humans evolved and were forced to adapt to periods without easy access to food, your body will invariably fail to run optimally when you continuously eat and ignore the age-honored traditions of taking time off from consuming food.

While I strongly advocate reducing your eating window to six to eight hours, the scientific literature is clear that the single most important step that you can implement is to stop eating at least three hours before bedtime.

Why? There are three major problems that arise when you eat too close to when you go to sleep for the night:

1. **It impairs your mitochondrial health.** The research[22] is abundantly clear on this. Your energy needs are the lowest when you are sleeping. When you give your body fuel when it does not need it, your mitochondrial ATP production system (which derives energy from the food you eat) backs up and you wind up directing much of that energy to being stored as fat. Excess fat produces an overabundance of reactive oxygen species (ROS), which will contribute to free radical damage of your cellular membranes, protein, and, most important, your DNA.

2. **It disrupts your circadian rhythm.** Your body, like all living creatures, is exquisitely designed to follow the rhythms of the sunrise and sunset. Every cell in your body has its own clock that tells your genes when to turn on and off, and every hormone, neurotransmitter, and organ follows a cycle where their functions change according to the time of day.

    Your circadian rhythm is what makes you alert during the day and sleepy at night, but it goes much deeper than these obvious functions—it also regulates your digestion, your cellular repair, and your muscle tone. Without a healthy circadian rhythm, it is very difficult to be healthy. And eating just before bed throws your circadian rhythm out of whack, causing its own cascade of ill effects.

3. **It decreases your ability to burn fat effectively.**
Once you are metabolically flexible and able to burn
fat for fuel, you will need to deplete your glycogen
(sugar) stores in your liver before your body transi-
tions to using your stored fats and creates ketones in
your liver for energy. When you eat close to bedtime
there typically isn't enough time to lower your liver
glycogen levels, and your sabotage the opportunity to
metabolically switch to burning fat.

Getting enough proper sleep at the right time is one of the
most important health strategies you can implement. If you don't
believe this, then I would strongly recommend you read Dr. Matthew Walker's recent book *Why We Sleep*. It will help you more
fully appreciate the massive health benefits that occur when you
give your body sufficient sleep. It will also help you understand
the dangers of not getting proper rest.

Every organ in your body requires rest, including all your
organs of digestion. According to Dr. Panda, these organs need
even more than the eight hours of rest they get with a healthy
night's sleep. Many organs need at least 12 hours of not pro-
cessing food so that they can repair themselves. As Dr. Panda
explains, "Just like you cannot repair a highway when the traffic
is still flowing, you cannot completely repair your gut if you just
keep on eating into your rest time."

Dr. Panda has done research on humans and on mice and
has found in both instances that restricting the eating window
to 12 hours or less kicks off a host of health benefits *even without*
ensuring that the food the subjects eat is nutrient-dense. While
of course I advocate eating nutrient-dense food, what's remarkable is that Dr. Panda's research shows that if you eat healthy
food *at the wrong time*, it can be just as detrimental as junk food.

And the opposite is also true. Even if you eat *poor-quality food*
in a time-restricted eating window, you will get benefits. In the
mice experiments, Dr. Panda took a group of mice born to the
same mother in the same room (so that their weight and their
population of gut bacteria were as close as possible) and divided

them into two groups: One group was fed the typical high-carb, high-sugar diet so many Americans eat, where they could eat whenever they wanted. The other group got the same diet and the same number of calories, but they were only allowed to eat those calories during a window of between eight and 12 hours a day. The time-restricted group was protected from obesity, diabetes, cardiovascular disease, systemic inflammation, high cholesterol, and other diseases that the non-time-restricted group fell prey to.

Even more important, when Dr. Panda and his researchers took overweight mice and restricted their feeding window to somewhere between 8 and 10 hours, they could reverse many of those same diseases. Dr. Panda and his colleagues also did a pilot study in which overweight volunteers ate only during a 10- to 11-hour window for 16 weeks. At the end of the intervention, the participants reported significant improvements in sleep satisfaction, energy levels, and hunger at bedtime. They also lost weight and kept it off for a year.

So the best first step into the fasting world that you can take is to stop eating at least three hours before you go to bed. Once that is a regular part of your daily routine—and generally it takes about a month to incorporate a new habit—you can move on to the next step, which is restricting your eating to a 12-hour window.

Think of eating only during a 12-hour window just like brushing your teeth—it's something you do on a daily basis that helps you maintain your current level of health. You may not be able to completely reverse disease by eating within a 12-hour window, but you won't be contributing to disease either. Just make sure that three of those hours when you are not eating happen just before bed. So if you go to bed at 11 P.M., have your last bite of food at 8 P.M. and then don't eat your first morsel until 8 A.M. the following morning.

When you overeat, eat primarily carbohydrates, or eat close to bedtime, your body produces far more ROS than when you periodically take a break from food and prioritize eating healthier foods such as high-quality fats and non-starchy, low-carb vegetables. When you fast, your mitochondria are freed up from constantly fighting off free radicals (since burning fat creates far fewer harmful ROS than burning sugar). They become healthier and can do their job more effectively and efficiently. They also get better at repairing themselves and taking themselves out of commission should they become damaged.

Incorporating KetoFasting into your life helps to address the primary reasons why you get sick in the first place. Going without food for a period of time provides the ultimate opportunity for the reversal of the consequences I've just listed, and gives you a chance to let your overfed and overburdened body take steps to restore its own health.

In the face of the current unprecedented epidemics of disease caused by dietary excess and chemical exposure, it makes sense that the ancient healing method of fasting is beginning to make intuitive sense to many people.

Before we look into what current research says about the benefits of fasting, let's first take a look at how fasting has been used throughout human history to support all manner of important aims beyond just health promotion. I think you'll be surprised and comforted to learn just what a long and important track record fasting has to support the strength and evolution of the human race.

SUMMARY

- Half of all Americans—that's 164 million people—have at least one chronic disease. While Western medicine is good at diagnosing these diseases, it falls short at providing information that helps prevent them from happening in the first place—or reversing them.

- Dietary changes over the past 100 years have contributed to the rise of chronic disease; this increase is likely related to the consumption of industrially processed omega-6 fats, a reduction in healthy saturated fats, and an overreliance on carbohydrate-rich grains and sugars, in addition to rarely going more than a few hours without food, other than while asleep.

- Our food supply and environment have become progressively more contaminated with harmful chemicals—from food additives, synthetic fertilizers, pesticides, and electromagnetic fields.

- Other factors contributing to this rise in disease prevalence include iron overload, changes in our microbiomes, and a rise in inflammation.

- All of these external disruptions have contributed to impaired mitochondrial health, which then kicks off a cascade of physiological events that can impair your body's ability to fight disease.

CHAPTER 2

THE HISTORY
OF FASTING

I know that fasting can seem like it's yet another diet fad in the vein of the low-cholesterol, low-fat, and gluten-free crazes that have swept through the public consciousness over the past few decades. Yet it is a tradition and a healing mechanism that is as old as humankind itself. In fact, fasting played a crucial role in early human survival. When you engage in it, you are participating in an activity that is woven into your very DNA and that has been practiced by your ancestors for millennia.

Fasting began simply as part of life. Evolutionary biologists speculate that we have had inconsistent access to food since our species began.[1] Even with the initial development of agricultural practices approximately 10,000 years ago and their gradual refinement over the centuries, food access remained unpredictable. It is only within the past 150 years that humans have achieved the high level of food predictability that we enjoy today, where we have the technology to not only grow the food but also refrigerate and transport it over long distances.

Evolutionarily speaking, 150 years is a mere blip in comparison to human ancestral time in which we, as a species, developed the metabolic flexibility to be able to produce ketones from fat when glucose supplies are low and enter a fat-burning state known as ketosis. It's this flexibility that enables our species to survive without food.

There are several evolutionary theories that attempt to explain how periodic food scarcity throughout human evolution shaped our ability to store fat,[2] but there are fewer theories on how it contributed to our efficient utilization of that fat to produce ketones that fuel the brain and other organs. Regardless, we simply aren't genetically and biochemically adapted to be able to eat continuously—as most of us have for the past century—and remain healthy. Now that we can walk over to the fridge or stop at any drive-through, we rarely get the opportunity to produce ketones, because our glucose and insulin levels remain high. Fasting is more than just a matter of necessity: it is a way for us to create conditions that contributed to the survival of our species.

> *"Fasting is the oldest dietary intervention in the world. . . . It is not just the latest and greatest, but the tried and true."*
>
> — DR. JASON FUNG, AUTHOR OF
> THE COMPLETE GUIDE TO FASTING

A look at the history of fasting shows that humans have been fasting not just because we sometimes didn't have a choice but because periodically going without foods provides a wide variety of other benefits, whether they are spiritual, political, religious, or therapeutic.[3, 4, 5]

(If you would like to take a deeper dive into fasting's history, *Fasting: An Exceptional Human Experience* by Randi Fredricks is the most comprehensive survey on fasting throughout human history published to date.)

RELIGIOUS FASTING

Religious fasting is documented in the sacred texts of every major religion, including, but not limited to:

- **Judaism.** The Hebrew Bible originated around 500 B.C.E. and its references to fasting have had a profound influence on the practice in Judaism. The Talmud, another sacred Jewish text written around 300 B.C.E., references several communal fasting days, including Yom Kippur and Tisha B'Av, which are day-long dry fasts. The Essenes, an ancient ascetic Jewish community, fasted on water for 40 days once per year to purify their bodies and develop a closer relationship with God.

    Jewish communities today traditionally fast during times of great upheaval, as an expression of mourning and gratitude, and in preparation for divine revelations. They also use fasting to commemorate meaningful life events, to repent, to honor the death of a loved one, and as an act of supplication. Fasting is obligatory after the age of 13 for boys and 12 for girls, but the ill as well as pregnant and breast-feeding women are not expected to fast. Fasting is also used as a method of transformation and to enhance spiritual awareness in Jewish mystical traditions, such as Kabbalah.

- **Christianity.** Fasting has been practiced in most Christian denominations including Anglicanism, Roman Catholicism, Greek Catholicism, Eastern Orthodoxy, and Oriental Orthodox churches to repent; to purify body, mind, and soul; to enhance prayer; and to overcome desires that are obstacles to one's relationship with God. The Bible, which originated in the early first millennium, makes reference to various fasts, the most famous of which are the 40-day fasts undertaken by Jesus and Moses.

Fasts mentioned in the Bible include partial fasts that involve abstaining from selected dietary items or meals, normal fasts that involve abstaining from all food and drink with the exception of water (i.e., water-only fasts), absolute fasts that involve abstaining from all food and drink (i.e., dry fasts), and supernatural fasts like the one undertaken by Moses when he survived for 40 days without eating or drinking. The Lenten fast, which is a 40-day partial fast in honor of the 40-day fast Jesus undertook in the desert, is perhaps the most well-known fast in Christianity. It is observed by both the Catholic and Eastern Orthodox churches, although other churches have similar 40-day fasting periods.

- **Islam.** The Koran, which originated around 600 C.E., provides instructions on three types of fasts: ritual fasting done on specific days in order to honor someone; penitent fasting done to repent or as self-sacrifice; and ascetic fasting that is undertaken to experience humility.

    Fasting during the holy month of Ramadan is obligatory for every physically and emotionally healthy adult who is not traveling. During this time, Muslims join together in abstaining from food, drink, and sexual relations between dawn and sunset, which is a form of time-restricted eating. Fasting more than every other day is not encouraged outside of the month of Ramadan.

    Sufism is a mystical branch of Islam that has a strong tradition of fasting. In this tradition, fasting is considered an essential spiritual practice that strengthens love, humility, patience, and gratitude, as well as helping to control physical desires. Sufis fast during Ramadan but also during the 40-day retreat undertaken by initiates.

Rumi, one of history's best-known poets from the 13th century, was a Sufi as well as a staunch practitioner and advocate of fasting. Of going without food, he wrote, "Fast and see the strength of the spirit reveal itself." Rumi also espoused fasting as a catalyst for creativity, as evidenced by this excerpt from one of his poems: "There's a hidden sweetness in the stomach's emptiness. / We are lutes, no more, no less. / If the soundbox is stuffed full of anything, no music comes. / If brain and belly are burning clean with fasting, every moment a new song comes out of the fire."

- **Buddhism.** Buddhism originated from the foundational teachings of the Buddha around 500 B.C.E. and is the largest religion in Asia. According to accounts of the life of the Buddha in the early texts (known as *sutras*), the Buddha (then called Siddhartha Gautama) began a spiritual life of renunciation by practicing severe asceticism for six years in which he denied his bodily needs, including the need for nourishment. Although he made progress along the spiritual path, he eventually realized that extreme asceticism was not enabling him to reach ultimate liberation and that physical strength was necessary to continue his path. After nourishing his body from a bowl of rice porridge, he spent the night in meditation and finally attained supreme enlightenment. The Buddha then went on to promote the middle way that did not involve severe ascetic practices such as denying the body food, but rather encouraged moderation, such as not eating after noon, which many Theravada monastics continue to do to this day.[6] Devout laypeople also refrain from eating after noon on special days of observance called Uposatha.

  Some Buddhist practitioners later adopted more rigorous fasting practices than those advocated by the Buddha himself. For example, in the Tibetan tradition, fasting is used in practices such as

Nyungne in which the practitioner eats the morning meal on the first day and then does not eat or speak the rest of that day, or at all on the second day, with the intention of purification of the body, mind, and spirit. Another fasting practice in the Tibetan tradition is Ningne, a half-day fast with the objective of avoiding reincarnation into the lower realms. For lay practitioners, fasting is often observed by forgoing particular food groups, such as meat. Fasting in Buddhism is used as a way to practice non-attachment, self-discipline, and, in some traditions, nonviolence.

- **Jainism.** The Jains engage in some of the most ardent fasting practices of any religion. The Jain fasting rituals are defined in the sacred books collectively called the Agamas (Aagam), which are dated as early as the 5th century B.C.E. In these texts, fasting is named the supreme spiritual practice.[7, 8] The aim of fasting for Jains is to practice nonviolence, diminish desires, repent, and purify body and mind—all of which ultimately dissolve karma.

  Jains practice several types of fasting, including abstention from all food and water, eating less than is needed, limiting the number of food items eaten, and giving up favorite foods. Jains also participate in so-called great fasts, in which the consumption of food is stopped for up to several months, and, more rarely, Santhara (or Sallekhana), a ritualistic fast to the death, which follows a strict code and is more similar to euthanasia than suicide.

- **Taoism.** Taoism dates its origins to a figure named Lao-tzu, who purportedly lived in the 6th century B.C.E. and composed the famous Tao Te Ching. Taoism places a strong emphasis on body cultivation for spiritual attainment, perhaps more so than any other major religion. This is based on the Taoist belief that everything in existence, including the human body, is made up of the same vital substance, qi (or chi). Self-cultivation practices such as breathing exercises, nutrition, and fasting (among many others) can augment, balance, nourish, and harmonize qi, and thus form the basis of human health. As qi is transformed, the body itself is transformed, leading first to the restoration of health, then to longevity, and ultimately (at the furthest extreme) to immortality.[9]

The most detailed and lengthy collection of religious dietary practices in the Taoist canon is found in the *Taishang Lingbao Wufuxu*, which was written between 100 and 400 C.E. It describes three levels of dietary asceticism.[10] At the first level, one begins by supplementing a normal or decreased diet with vegetables, herbs, and minerals with specific energetic resonances (forms of qi) that begin to transform the body. At the second level, one shifts from supplementing to actually replacing a normal diet with small amounts of these substances. At the third level, one engages in extensive fasting practices, consuming no food or water and ingesting cosmic qi through specialized breathing and visualization practices. Different benefits correspond to each level of rigor. First and foremost is curing the "hundred diseases" (*baibing*)—that is, all disease. This is followed by perfecting one's health, which involves restoring eyesight and hearing, strengthening bones and muscles, rejuvenating the complexion, as well as restoring graying hair and teeth. From that point, continuing to follow the increasingly rigorous protocol leads to extraordinary attainments such as clairvoyance, clairaudience, becoming impervious to cold and heat, and developing the ability to fly. Lastly, the body itself becomes spiritualized, leading to extreme longevity (400 to 40,000 years) or even immortality.[11]

HUNGER STRIKES

Hunger strikes are a political form of fasting. They are used as a form of nonviolent resistance in which the participant voluntarily forgoes food (and sometimes water), usually with the intention of bringing attention to an alleged personal or societal injustice.[12, 13] It is very rare that a person who is hunger striking will fast to the death.

One of the earliest accounts of political fasting appeared in the *Ramayana*, an ancient Indian epic poem that was composed beginning in the 5th century B.C.E.[14] The story goes that Bharata, the brother of Rama, intended to fast to the death to protest Rama's exile from the kingdom. However, Bharata never completed his fast because Rama intervened and the fast was stopped. There are also accounts of hunger strikes in pre-Christian Ireland, as far back as 1,500 years ago, with a tradition termed *troscadh* or *cealachan*, in which a person who felt wronged by another would fast at the alleged wrongdoer's doorstep.[15] This strategy apparently worked because it was considered a grave dishonor to allow a person to die at one's doorstep, and if the faster died, then the accused wrongdoer would have to pay the debts of the deceased.

Although hunger strikes are still commonly used to protest a variety of alleged injustices, the most publicized political fasts occurred in the 20th century, including those by the suffragettes in the early 1900s and Irish political prisoners in the 1980s. And then, of course, there is Gandhi.

The most famous political faster is the Indian activist Mahatma Gandhi (1869–1948), who engaged in 17 hunger strikes between 1913 and 1948, the longest fast being 21 days.[16] Gandhi fasted to protest societal injustices and violence, as well as to promote unity between Hindus and Muslims. Although Gandhi undertook fasts in which he intended to fast to the death for the cause he was protesting, he never fasted to that extreme because his demands were typically met long before that point was reached. Fasting was also a spiritual practice for Gandhi, as he wrote, "The light of the world will illuminate within you when you fast and purify yourself."

THERAPEUTIC FASTING

The end goal of therapeutic fasting is physical health, though there may well be spiritual benefits, too. There is evidence that ancient Greek scholars, including Plato, Plutarch, and Hippocrates, promoted the use of therapeutic fasting more than 2,000 years ago.[17]

Plato wrote, "I fast for greater physical and mental efficiency." Plutarch declared, "Instead of using medicine, better fast today." And Hippocrates said about fasting, "Everyone has a doctor in him; we just have to help him in his work. The natural healing force within each one of us is the greatest force in getting well. To eat when you are sick is to feed your sickness." Although these early civilizations and enormously influential thinkers espoused fasting as a more powerful alternative to the science of medicine for healing, suggesting that patients go without food in order to promote health has mostly occurred only on the fringes of the medical community. While this has very recently begun to change, there have been a few people and movements that have kept the flame alive until now.

In the 15th century, the physician Philippus Paracelsus—one of the three fathers of Western medicine—referenced the body's natural healing mechanisms and fasting's ability to stimulate them when he wrote, "Fasting is the greatest remedy—the physician within." Benjamin Franklin also heralded fasting's healing abilities in the late 1700s when he wrote, "The best of all medicines is resting and fasting." While Franklin wasn't a medical professional, he was a significant and influential scientific thinker.

I learned a lot about the history of fasting in America from Dr. Alan Goldhamer, who has overseen the water-only fasts of more than 16,000 patients at his TrueNorth Health Center in Northern California, and who consulted on this book. The form of therapeutic fasting Goldhamer practices had its beginnings in the Natural Hygiene Movement, which was started in 1811 by Isaac Jennings (1788–1874), regarded as the first physician in the U.S. to use therapeutic fasting and hygienic principles in lieu of medicinal drugs.[18] Sylvester Graham (1792–1851), a Presbyterian minister and creator of the graham cracker, helped popularize Jennings' teachings by staunchly advocating fasting as well as a vegetarian diet, pure water, sunshine, clean air, abstinence from intoxicants, exercise, emotional poise, and rest.

Other American physicians followed in the hygienic tradition, and many graduated as medical doctors from eclectic medical schools and published various works on lifestyle, diet, and fasting. Although the teaching and practice of Natural Hygiene or "nature cure" continued at various clinics over the next century, it fell out of practice with the rising predominance of more conventional medicinal approaches.

Then came an unexpected, successful fasting experience by Henry Tanner, M.D. In 1877, Dr. Tanner was a respected, middle-aged physician living in Duluth, Minnesota. He had suffered for years with rheumatism and had consulted with several fellow physicians, all of whom considered his case to be "hopeless." He also suffered from asthma, which chronically disrupted his sleep. He spent his waking hours in constant pain.

Tanner had been taught in medical school that humans could live only 10 days without food, and in this knowledge he found solace. He determined that he would simply starve himself to death. As he stated later, "Life to me under the circumstances was not worth living . . . and I had made up my mind to rest from physical suffering in the arms of death." But fate had an agreeable surprise for Dr. Tanner. By unwittingly invoking a constellation of health-promoting responses associated with water-only fasting, he rapidly recovered.

By the fifth day of his fast, Tanner was able to begin to sleep more peacefully. By the 11th day, he reported feeling "as well as in my youthful days." Fully expecting that by this point he should be near death, he asked a fellow physician, Dr. Moyer, to examine him. Not surprisingly, Dr. Moyer was amazed.

According to Tanner's recollection, Moyer told him, "You ought to be at death's door, but you certainly look better than I ever saw you before." Tanner continued to fast, under Dr. Moyer's supervision, for an additional 31 days—a total of 42 days in all.

When fellow physicians heard his story, which was sensationalized in the press, they responded with disbelief and intense criticism. Though widely rebuked as a fraud, Tanner at least had the last laugh. After his fast, Tanner had no symptoms of asthma, rheumatism, or chronic pain and lived a full life until he died at age 90.

In the decades after Tanner's experience, a few proponents of the Natural Hygiene Movement kept the knowledge and practice of therapeutic fasting alive in the United States, which may explain why, in 1903, Mark Twain wrote in his work *My Debut as a Literary Person*, "A little starvation can really do more for the average sick man than can the best medicines and the best doctors."

But it wasn't until 1911, when Herbert M. Shelton, N.D., D.C. (1895–1985),[19] became interested in hygienic principles and began educating himself with literature written by popular hygienists of the time, that the Natural Hygiene Movement truly began to experience a resurgence. Shelton later studied under fasting authorities at MacFadden's College (in Chicago), Crane's Sanatorium (in Elmhurst, Illinois), and Crandall's Health School (in York, Pennsylvania). In 1928, he founded a fasting institution and health school that provided services for more than 40 years. He also published numerous books on fasting and Natural Hygiene and developed a strict fasting protocol that specified consuming only water, avoiding enemas, exercise, or treatments, and observing complete rest, which is the foundation of the therapeutic fasting protocol used by the Northern California–based TrueNorth Health Center, which is the largest water fasting clinic in North America.[20]

In 1949, Dr. Shelton, along with William Esser, N.D., D.C., Christopher Gian-Cursio, N.D., D.C., and Gerald Benesh, N.D., D.C., formed the American Natural Hygiene Society, which is now the National Health Association (NHA). NHA is a lay organization dedicated to preserving the tenets of Natural Hygiene. In 1978, the International Association of Hygienic Physicians (IAHP) was formed to promote the professional use of Natural Hygiene. IAHP continues to this day, and organizes clinical training and examination to certify clinicians in therapeutic fasting. The TrueNorth Health Center is currently the only medically supervised, water-only fasting center in the U.S. with IAHP certification.

Although fasting did begin returning to prominence in the medical realm throughout the 20th century, that time also witnessed a period of remarkable medical innovation in surgical techniques, radiation therapies, and new "miracle" drugs that still mostly drowned out a larger awareness and appreciation of the self-healing mechanisms that are unleashed during fasting.

In the early part of the 21st century, something extraordinary is occurring: After decades of collective awe of modern medicine and its purveyors, a strong undercurrent of disillusionment has begun to appear. With it came the beginnings of a philosophical revolution that is leading health science in a promising new direction.

This new direction centers on the realization that health and healing are best supported when the biological roots of our nature are better understood and respected. This philosophical approach is based on the awareness that health and healing are natural processes, and that the body seeks to be healthy by default as long as we provide it with what it requires.

As a result, the focus of attention has increasingly shifted away from the conventional medical emphasis on drugs and surgery toward an exploration of the approaches and strategies necessary to unleash and enhance these natural processes—exactly as fathers of medicine Hippocrates and Paracelsus espoused two millennia ago.

Now we'll look at the benefits of fasting—borne from a history of hundreds of thousands of years—as well as more recent scientific findings that fasting offers extraordinary potential for health and healing. For some conditions, it appears to be the most effective treatment available.

With such clear and convincing evidence to guide them and substantial cost savings to motivate them, it is my sincere desire that individuals, medical schools, hospital systems, unions, and insurance companies choose to encourage and support the use of fasting for those they serve. In doing so, they could make available to the millions of sick and suffering patients the most profound health rediscovery of our time: the understanding that fasting allows the body to heal itself without the risk and excess cost associated with conventional medical care and drug use.

SUMMARY

- Fasting is a healing tradition that has existed as long as the human race has existed.

- Humans' ability to burn ketones (small water-soluble fats) and glucose for fuel has been crucial to our species' survival.

- Fasting has been an integral part of many of the world's religions for its purifying abilities and spiritual benefits.

- Fasting—in the form of hunger strikes—has also been used to further political causes, including by Gandhi, who undertook 17 hunger strikes during his life.

- Fasting for better health was heralded by Plato, Plutarch, and Hippocrates more than 2,000 years ago.

- The tradition of therapeutic fasting in the United States was codified in 1811 by Isaac Jennings, the founder of the Natural Hygiene Movement.

CHAPTER 3

THE MECHANISMS OF FASTING

As discussed, fasting is one of the oldest dietary interventions in the world. Modern science confirms that it can have a profoundly beneficial influence on health for all different types of creatures—humans, animals, and even simple organisms all respond to a lack of nutrients with physiological adaptations that clearly seem to improve condition, and even lifespan. For example, *E. coli* (bacteria), *S. cerevisiae* (yeast), and *C. elegans* (roundworm) grown without nutrients survive longer than when they are fed a nutrient-rich diet.

Why is fasting such an important health-promoting strategy? Essentially, it is a positive stressor to your body. But what exactly does it do for your physiology that makes it so beneficial? Let's take a look at the processes it initiates.

REDUCES INSULIN RESISTANCE

Insulin resistance is one of the most dangerous and widespread health conditions there is. It is estimated that 80 percent of

Americans, maybe even more, have it. This may seem high, but in Dr. Joseph Kraft's book, *The Diabetes Epidemic and You,* he describes a highly sensitive test to measure insulin resistance. It is performed very similarly to an oral glucose tolerance test, however insulin levels are measured in addition to glucose. When Dr. Kraft did his analysis, he found that 80 percent of Americans were insulin resistant, and that was over 15 years ago. Insulin resistance is the precursor to diabetes, obesity, heart and neurodegenerative diseases, cancer, and many other chronic diseases that are also epidemic. The good news is that fasting is one of the most effective ways to restore normal sensitivity to your insulin receptors.

Insulin is the primary hormone that tells your body whether to store energy or burn it. When you eat—particularly when you eat the typical high-carb, heavily processed foods that most Americans eat at all hours of the day—your blood glucose levels become elevated to unhealthy ranges. Your body then increases your insulin in an effort to lower those glucose levels.

Sadly this results in an enormously foolish medical strategy that many physicians use to treat tens of millions of diabetics— they frequently put type 2 diabetics on insulin in an effort to lower their blood sugar. What they fail to realize is that higher insulin levels, and secondary insulin resistance, are a far more serious issue than elevated glucose.

The way to lower insulin *and* glucose and to treat insulin resistance is to lower your carbohydrate intake and become metabolically flexible, as co-author of *The Complete Guide to Fasting* and a nephrologist (kidney specialist) in Canada, so eloquently demonstrated in his 2018 case report published in the *British Medical Journal.* In this report, Dr. Fung was able to use intermittent fasting to reverse insulin resistance and resolve type 2 diabetes for three patients who had their diabetes for 10 to 25 years. All were taking insulin.[1] One result of insulin resistance is that you gain weight because higher levels of insulin signal your body to store energy as fat. Another result is that the receptors for insulin in your cells begin to get desensitized, so you need to release more and more insulin in order to move the glucose out of your bloodstream and into your cells. As a result of the insulin resistance, your body is in constant fat-storing mode.

The key to breaking this cycle is to have sustained low insulin levels, which is why fasting can be so tremendously beneficial. When you take a break from eating, your blood glucose level falls, and as your glucose level falls, your pancreas produces less and less insulin, as it simply isn't needed. In fact, *fasting lowers insulin more powerfully than any other strategy* we know of. And when your insulin levels fall, your body gets the cue to release energy so you will start to burn your fat stores. It also allows your insulin receptors to regain their sensitivity so that when you enter the refeeding phase of your fast, your body won't need to use as much insulin to maintain healthy blood glucose levels. That's when insulin resistance resolves, and you begin to recover your health.

If you engage in Peak Fasting or time restricted eating for at least 16 hours, you will tend to deplete the glycogen stores in your liver.

If, like most Americans, you have been eating a high-carb diet for many years, it might take you longer to deplete your glycogen stores and lower your glucose and insulin levels, but persistence will pay off and you will eventually do it. Once you are able to deplete your glycogen levels, your insulin resistance will soon resolve, as will your risk for virtually all chronic, degenerative diseases. The timing of the next step will vary from person to person, but eventually your insulin resistance will resolve and you will regain your metabolic flexibility and once again be able to burn your fat stores effectively. Once you have resolved your insulin resistance and regained your metabolic flexibility, your liver will start transforming your stored body fat—in a process known as lipolysis—into ketones and releasing them into your bloodstream to be used as energy by your most metabolically active tissues, including your brain and heart.

Note that the time needed to achieve your goal of regaining your ability to burn fat as your primary fuel will vary greatly, based on your individual circumstances. If you are undergoing a medically supervised water fast for a specific health condition, this process generally takes two to three days. If you're following a cyclical ketogenic diet or a supported fast, it will typically take a few weeks. If you are more than 50 pounds overweight and have been metabolically inflexible for a number of years, it could take several weeks or even months.

AUTOPHAGY

Another magnificent healing mechanism that fasting triggers is the process of autophagy. *Auto* in Greek means "self," and *phagy* means "to eat," so autophagy refers to your body digesting its own damaged cells. It is a vital cleanout process—the equivalent of taking out the trash—that detoxifies your cells and recycles the parts of the organelles within them that are no longer needed, so that your cells behave more youthfully. Autophagy also destroys foreign invaders such as viruses, bacteria, and other pathogens.

A similar process, apoptosis, is when the *entire* cell is recycled. When apoptosis is impaired, your risk for cancer increases dramatically because your ability to remove damaged cells is impaired. That is why fasting is so useful as an adjunctive strategy to not only prevent cancer, but also help treat it.

Autophagy naturally slows down with age, and this decrease is known to contribute to a wide variety of diseases, including Alzheimer's and Parkinson's. By activating autophagy, or repairing the mechanism in cases where dysfunction has set in, researchers believe neurodegenerative diseases such as Alzheimer's and Parkinson's can be improved, as the autophagy process will naturally clear out harmful proteins. Without this process, your cells will eventually become overwhelmed with toxins and debris, which radically impairs their ability to function properly and frequently leads to premature cell death.

There is a wide variety of ways to boost autophagy, but the most effective way by far is to fast. When you allow your body to go without food, your cells will trigger your autophagy switch as part of the mechanism that enables it to adapt to your lack of food and still produce the energy your body needs.[2] Then, during the refeeding phase, your growth hormone increases, boosting the building of new proteins and cells. In other words, fasting and then breaking the fast reactivates and speeds up your body's natural renewal cycle.

This is very similar to exercise, as exercise itself typically causes muscle and cellular damage from which your body recovers and builds stronger muscles and tissues. We all know that exercise is vital for good health and without it you will wither away. And we also know that if you overexercise, you can cause serious damage. Optimal recovery is key to maximizing the benefits of exercise.

Fasting works exactly the same way. If you fast continuously without recovery phases, you will hurt your body. The magic of fasting actually occurs in the refeeding phase when you build yourself a new, healthier body.

Ways to Stimulate Autophagy

Exercise intensely (not too much). Every other day, do 30 minutes of high-intensity interval training or resistance training. The acute stress of exercise triggers autophagy much in the same way as fasting by stimulating a metabolic pathway called PGC-1 alpha that also increases mitochondrial biogenesis.

Activate adenosine monophosphate-activated protein kinase (AMPK). AMPK is an enzyme that stimulates mitochondrial autophagy (mitophagy) and mitochondrial biogenesis as well as five other critically important pathways: insulin, leptin, mammalian target of rapamycin (mTOR), insulin-like growth factor 1, and peroxisome proliferator-activated receptor gamma co-activator 1-alpha (PPAR⌧). It also increases nerve growth factor and helps protect against the type of oxidative stress that leads to Parkinson's disease. Your AMPK levels naturally decline with increasing age.

Following a cyclical ketogenic diet will help you maintain healthy AMPK levels. Eating too much unhealthy fat and not enough healthy fat, and getting insufficient amounts of polyphenolic flavonoids (antioxidants) will inhibit AMPK activity. Most people know about the 220 minus your age formula to determine maximum heart rate, but to increase your AMPK levels and autophagy, it's better to use cardio exercises that keep your heart rate at a constant 180 minus your age. It will also help propel you into the fat-burning zone.

Regular exposure to cold temperatures has also been shown to increase AMPK; it also activates longevity proteins called sirtuins. They normally require a co-factor, nicotinamide adenine dinucleotide, or NAD+ (with the plus sign indicating the oxidized form of the compound), to become activated; however, exposure to cold is an alternate way to activate sirtuins. Cold exposure is ideally done after an infrared sauna by jumping in a cool pool (approximately 65 degrees), or you can alternate between cold and hot showers for 1-minute cycles, for a total of 10 minutes, ending on cold.

Insulin resistance is also a powerful inhibitor of AMPK. So, keeping this enzyme activated through proper diet is another important factor for maintaining healthy autophagy. You can also activate AMPK through dietary supplements. These supplements also benefit your mitochondrial function and health:

- Pyrroloquinoline quinone (PQQ)
- Berberine
- EGCG from green tea or apple peels
- Curcumin
- Apigenin, a flavone found in parsley and chamomile
- Anthocyanins, found in blueberries
- Quercetin, found in many fruits and vegetables
- Resveratrol or its better absorbed cousin, pterostilbene
- Apple cider vinegar
- CoQ10 or ubiquinol
- Cinnamon
- Omega-3 from fish or krill
- Astragalus

FREE STEM CELL TRANSPLANT!

As important as autophagy is for clearing out dysfunctional or diseased cell components, it's only half the battle. You also want to trigger new, healthy cells and cell components to be manufactured, and this is where stem cells come in.

There is plenty of buzz about stem cells. Stem cells are such powerful regenerators that people undergo stem cell transplantation for a variety of reasons, but primarily in hopes of spurring their body into healing itself. However, they can be very expensive, typically costing thousands of dollars in treatment. A particularly fascinating aspect of fasting is that it improves your body's stem cell production. As an adult your stem cells are undifferentiated, or not committed to a specific cell type, and are found in tissues and organs that are used by your body to renew itself. The primary role of these cells is to maintain and repair your tissues where they are found.[3]

Apart from the high cost, a drawback to stem cell transplants is that when you inject stem cells, the stem cells lack the program that tells them what to do. But when you fast, the refeeding phase automatically provides instructions to the stem cells you already have, telling them to rebuild everything that is now missing. For this reason it is certainly far less expensive and perhaps even more effective to activate your stem cells naturally, via fasting and refeeding, than by having stem cells injected.

Researchers at the University of Southern California have found that fasting reduces levels of insulin-like growth factor 1 (IGF-1), a hormone whose pathway regulates growth and aging, and the enzyme PKA,[4] which is linked to the orchestration of stem cell renewal. As IGF-1 and PKA shut down, stem cell regeneration switches on.

Additionally, research funded by the National Institutes of Health recently documented that mice that fasted for only one day actually doubled their regenerative capacity.[5] **They found that one single fast improved intestinal stem cell function in both young and aged mice, by boosting fat metabolism.** Intestinal stem cells are responsible for maintaining the lining of the intestine, which typically renews itself every five days. When an injury or infection occurs, stem cells are necessary for repairing any damage. As people age, the regenerative abilities of these intestinal stem cells decline, so it takes longer for the intestine to recover. Intestinal stem cells are the workhorses of the intestine, giving rise to more stem cells and to all the various differentiated cell types of the intestine.

It appears that using fats for energy preserves the health and function of intestinal stem cells, and that the ability to break down and use fats for energy is impaired in older individuals—*unless they fast*. Of course, mice have a much higher metabolic rate than humans, so one day of fasting for a mouse is equal to several days for humans. Nonetheless, these results are very impressive for a variety of reasons related to stem cell activation.

HAPPY STEM CELLS RUN ON FAT

The NIH researchers working with mice discovered a very interesting phenomenon, where some period of fasting seemed to have beneficial effects on stem cells in both younger and older mice. But what mechanisms were at play? Through clever experimentation, they discovered that burning fats may be the cause of improved stem cell function in the fasting mice. When the researchers turned off fat metabolism through genetic engineering, they were able to block the benefits of fasting on the mice's intestinal stem cells.

The typical American diet gets about 60 to 70 percent of its energy from carbohydrates or sugar, about 20 percent from fat, and the remainder mostly from protein. What's really interesting is that when you fast, you start to derive much more energy from the breakdown of fat. The NIH study provided evidence that fasting induces a metabolic switch in the intestinal stem cells, from utilizing carbohydrates to burning fat. Interestingly, switching these cells to fat burning enhanced their function significantly. Which is to say, the researchers believe that when the mice were fasting, their intestinal stem cells (in both young and old mice) switched from utilizing carbohydrates to using fat as their primary energy source. This metabolic switch is what's driving an improvement in stem cell function.

Not only will your intestinal stem cells make the switch, but stem cells all over your body will do so as well. It will just take longer than one day because you are not a mouse.

DETOXIFICATION

As we've talked about, in today's world most of us are exposed to countless toxins on a nearly continuous basis, and so we have all of these toxins stored in the tissues of our body—primarily our fat. Research even shows that infants are now born with toxins in their cord blood—toxins absorbed from their mother.[6, 7]

Many of these chemicals are endocrine-disrupting, which means they alter the function of hormones, so even a relatively tiny amount of exposure can create a profoundly negative effect. For all of these reasons, detoxification is an important process that needs to be done on a regular basis if you are seeking optimal health.

Fasting is one of the most potent ways to remove toxins from your body. This is because when you are fasting and fat-adapted, your body is largely burning fat for fuel. To access this fat, your body breaks down your fat stores, a process known as lipolysis. Lipolysis will help mobilize the fat-soluble toxins stored in your fat. The more you access your fat stores for fuel, such as during fasting or time-restricted eating, the more the toxins will be mobilized and released from your tissues.

This is good news and bad news; the good news is that fasting will mobilize fat-soluble toxins, freeing them to be excreted through your sweat, urine, or feces. The bad news is, if you don't bind those toxins and facilitate their excretion by supporting your detoxification pathways, you *won't* actually excrete them. Instead, they most likely will be reabsorbed and remain in your body and continue to wreak havoc on your health.

I cover this process in much greater detail in Chapter 6, but I include it here because the detoxification that fasting triggers can be a major benefit, as long as you are careful to support the detoxification pathways, which is exactly what the KetoFast protocol is designed to do.

CIRCADIAN RHYTHMS

As we discussed in Chapter 1, your body's internal clock—known as your circadian rhythm—orchestrates nearly every process in your body, so when it is disrupted, a cascade of negative effects can happen. By taking a break from eating, you give your circadian rhythms a chance to normalize. In KetoFasting you will no longer interrupt your natural cycles by eating at times when your energy requirements and your insulin and glucose responses are at their lowest—primarily in the evening and at night.[8] This will help to stabilize many of your important systems, including your sleep and insulin sensitivity.

GUT HEALTH

The population of microbes that live in your gut—which is as distinct to you as your fingerprint—plays an enormous role in health and disease prevention. Your gut flora influences the function of various internal organs, such as your skin, lungs, breasts, and liver. Dozens of other conditions have been traced back to the influence of gut microbes as well, including obesity, depression, chronic fatigue syndrome, Parkinson's disease, and allergies,[9] just to name a few. One of the reasons for this is because a large part of your immune system is controlled by the health of your digestive system. When you disrupt your gut microbiome, you automatically impair your immune function, which can have far-reaching health consequences.

Your microbiome is largely influenced by your diet—both what you eat and when you eat it—and has a circadian rhythm of its own. When you fast, you help reset this rhythm and promote diversity in the types of microbes that reside in your gut. This then helps ward off all the diseases that are associated with poor gut health and improves the function of your immune system in general.

Fasting is also believed to help reduce gut permeability by stimulating a brain-gut pathway that enhances the integrity of your gut lining.[10] Increased gut permeability, also known as leaky gut, results when there's a disruption in the interconnections among the cells lining your intestines. Once the integrity of your intestinal lining is compromised, it allows toxic substances to enter your bloodstream.

Your body then releases a stream of inflammatory messengers to attack these "offenders," and you experience a significant increase in inflammation as a result. Your immune system may also become confused and begin to attack your own body as if it were your enemy—a hallmark of autoimmunity disorders. Fasting allows the junctures between the cells in your gut lining to heal and restore their integrity, which removes a major impediment to your overall health.

WEIGHT LOSS

It's probably not a surprise that dramatically reducing the number of calories you eat results in weight loss. But restricting your calories also lowers your insulin sensitivity, which is a primary controller of weight. When you fast, you lower your insulin levels so your body is no longer receiving the signal to store extra calories as fat. In fact, quite the opposite happens—your body begins accessing your fat stores and burning it as fuel. So the weight you lose as a result of regular fasting isn't just from water or muscle tissue; a large portion is from what you want to access, your fat stores.[11] It is particularly effective for reducing your visceral fat, which has been linked to cardiovascular disease.

If done correctly, fasting can also paradoxically raise your metabolic rate, which then further promotes weight loss and maintenance. This is very different from what happens when you merely cut calories. Prolonged calorie restriction alone is highly problematic, and why I don't recommend chronic ketosis. It is key to cycle in and out of ketosis once you have flipped your fat-burning switch and are able to burn fat for fuel. If you continue with long-term calorie restriction or uninterrupted ketosis, at some point your body will believe it's in starvation mode and downregulate your metabolism by decreasing your thyroid function.

Dr. Jason Fung has helped thousands of patients overcome their type 2 diabetes through fasting. According to his work, when you fast, your basal metabolic rate (the number of calories you need to burn to support normal function) actually goes *up by 10 percent.*

That's because fasting helps train your body to burn fat, which is typically available in plentiful supply, so your body doesn't feel the need to hold back on consuming the calories locked in that fat. It's like an all-you-can eat buffet, as it's estimated that the average person has tens of thousands of calories stored in their fat, as opposed to only 1,600 to 2,000 in their glycogen stores.[12] Burning fat gives you access to nearly unlimited energy stores, which means that you also feel much more energetic.

Best of all, you will preserve your muscle mass when fasting. Going without food actually downregulates protein catabolism (when your muscle tissue is consumed for fuel) and upregulates growth hormones and adrenaline, which preserves your muscles. So fasting helps you become leaner *and* stronger, exactly what you are looking for.

BRAIN FUNCTION

Fasting is an absolute boon to your brain health. This is in large part a result of your liver's ability to generate ketones again. Ketones are the form of fuel that your brain and heart prefer, as they produce far fewer harmful reactive oxygen species (ROS) than glucose, and have been shown to help reduce oxidative damage in the neurons of your neocortex.[13]

As a result, your brain can work more efficiently while incurring less damage. In fact, animal studies suggest that intermittent fasting can not only improve the ability of your brain to function, but also improve the cells in your brain through a process called neuroplasticity, and actually help you to learn more easily.[14] In addition to naturally supporting your ability to think and learn, there are other important benefits that fasting lends the brain:

- Ketones protect your brain cells that are exposed to oxidative stressors such as hydrogen peroxide, which is common in the brains of people with neurodegenerative diseases such as Alzheimer's and Parkinson's.[15]

- Ketones also increase the production of new mitochondria in your brain (mitochondrial biogenesis),[16] boosting the health and energy-producing capabilities of your brain cells.

- Less quantifiable but also important is the fact that fasting has been frequently reported to improve mental well-being by inducing feelings of mild euphoria.[17]

- Intermittent fasting has been shown to boost mood, improve memory, trigger the generation of new neurons, and lower the risk of aging-related cognitive decline.[18]

HEART FUNCTION

Heart disease is the leading cause of death in the U.S. Heart failure became an epidemic in the latter half of the 20th century[19] and continues to present an enormous threat to an ever-increasing percentage of the population. Fortunately, KetoFasting and the metabolic flexibility it brings can provide enormous benefits to the cells of your heart.[20]

Your heart cells have tremendous potential for metabolic flexibility, as they can use different energy sources, including fats, carbohydrates, ketones, and even amino acids to meet their high energy demand to sustain their pumping function.[21] Due to this metabolic flexibility, the heart's energy preference can rapidly change based on the presence of available fuels. Mitochondrial oxidative phosphorylation produces the majority of the high-energy phosphates needed to sustain the heart's pumping function.

Most people, including physicians (even cardiologists), are not aware that fats are the biggest contributor to mitochondrial oxidative metabolism in the heart.[22] Fats provide approximately 40 to 60 percent of the total energy produced in your heart, while the burning of glucose, ketones, and amino acids provides the remaining 20 to 40 percent. Ketones have a fine-tuning metabolic role that optimizes heart performance in varying nutrient states and protects the heart from inflammation and injury.[23]

Regularly incorporating healthy partial fasting into your life is one of the best ways I know of to support your body's innate maintenance and healing systems. In the next chapter, we'll look at different fasting techniques and philosophies so you can determine the approach that's right for you.

SUMMARY

- Appropriate partial fasting is a beneficial metabolic stressor, very similar to appropriate exercise.

- Partial fasting lowers insulin resistance more powerfully than any other method we currently know of.

- Partial fasting encourages autophagy, which recycles the parts of cells that are no longer needed—the equivalent of your cells taking out the trash—and apoptosis, which recycles entire cells that no longer function properly or are able to reproduce.

- Other ways to stimulate autophagy include intense exercise, implementing a cyclical ketogenic diet, and incorporating cold exposure into your regular routine.

- Partial fasting also improves your body's stem cell production, which triggers new, healthy cells to be manufactured.

- Other ways partial fasting improves your health is by helping your body liberate stored toxic chemicals, resetting your circadian rhythms, improving your gut health, lowering insulin resistance, promoting weight loss, and supporting optimal brain and heart function.

CHAPTER 4

THE DIFFERENT TYPES OF FASTING

There are nearly as many different ways to fast as there are ways to eat. Because there are so many different approaches, and so much information is available on the Internet on the best ways to fast, I want to give an overview here so that you will be better equipped to discern the right approach for you and better able to understand why I landed on the strategy that I call KetoFasting. I believe this strategy is suitable for most individuals.

There are three basic categories of fasting:

- **Intermittent fasting.** This will be a variation of eating with some form of fasting incorporated, whether that's on a daily, weekly, monthly, seasonal, or yearly basis. Intermittent fasting includes time-restricted eating (TRE). There are many different approaches to intermittent fasting, and I discuss the major ones below, but my choice (which I review in my book *Fat for Fuel*) is Peak Fasting, in which you limit the number of hours you eat your food to a restricted window of time.

That eating window is somewhere between six and eight hours. (More extreme restrictions, like reducing the window to four or even two hours, aren't typically necessary.) For example, you can eat a late breakfast and only consume food between the hours of 11 A.M. and 6 P.M. Or you can choose to have an early dinner, shifting your eating window to between 9 A.M. and 4 P.M. You should always stop eating at least three hours before you go to bed. This means you will go at least 16 to 18 hours without food. This time could extend to 20 or even 22 hours, but I have found that there is little to no benefit in extending an intermittent fast beyond 18 hours, especially if done on a long-term basis.

- **Partial fasting.** This is fasting longer than 24 hours while consuming 75 percent fewer calories than you normally do, usually for less than five days. KetoFasting is a very specific type of partial fasting in which you greatly reduce the number of calories you eat in a day to approximately 300 to 600, depending on your lean body mass, and eat only foods that will keep your body in a fasted state and help you process any fat-soluble toxins that might be released in your body during your fasting process (more on this in Chapters 7 and 8).

- **Water fasting.** This type of fasting is just as it sounds— you consume only water for the duration of the fast. No coffee, no teas, no MCT oils—just water. This is generally done for a specific therapeutic reason, especially for those with serious diseases. It can be a very powerful intervention and many may want to consider this approach, but it is an advanced technique.

In general, there's enormous fear around water fasting. Many believe their body will go into starvation mode, resulting in all sorts of muscle loss and metabolic catastrophes, not to mention having to struggle with unrelenting hunger for days on end. In

The Complete Guide to Fasting, Dr. Jason Fung explains that hunger doesn't consistently grow and grow and grow when you undertake a fast. Rather, it comes in waves. And my personal experience corroborates this.

There are many different ways you can incorporate water fasting into your dietary plan; however, I do not recommend you try water fasting on your own. I believe it should only be done with the supervision of a health-care provider who has extensive experience in therapeutic fasting or at a dedicated fasting facility. Multiple-day water fasting is a powerful intervention that is typically reserved for those with serious health problems. You can go to www.healthpromoting.com for a list of clinicians who are trained in this process.

THE STEALTH REASON YOU NEED TO BE CAREFUL WHEN WATER FASTING

Prior to writing this book, I believed that water fasting was the most powerful metabolic intervention I had ever encountered in my nearly four decades of clinical practice. Then I studied Dr. Bryan Walsh's outstanding course on detoxification and realized that there is indeed a dark side to water fasting that makes it a far less than ideal fasting strategy for the bulk of the population.

So, what is the problem with water fasting?

The major concern is that more than 85,000 chemicals have been created in the past century, and their presence in our environment, our food, and the products we use every day makes exposure to them virtually unavoidable. To help you understand how pervasive our exposure to harmful chemicals is—as well as how manufacturers go to great lengths to hide information about the toxicity of their ingredients—watch the 2015 documentary *Stink!* (As I write this, it is available for streaming on Netflix.) It will enlighten you on how common these exposures are.

Most of these chemicals are fat-soluble toxins; as a result, when your body is exposed to them, they are stored in your fat cells. The more fat you have, the more of these toxins you are likely storing.

Examples of some of these toxins include:

- **Mold toxins.** These are ubiquitous in the environment. Chronic exposure induces cancer through a variety of mechanisms. Not everyone is susceptible to sickness from mold, but mold expert Ritchie Shoemaker, M.D., estimates that 25 percent of all people cannot adequately detoxify mold,[1] which means that mold toxins, or mycotoxins, can accumulate in some people and cause symptoms or disease. Some molds, like aflatoxin, have been linked to cancer.

- **Heavy metals**, such as mercury, arsenic, lead, cadmium, and others, are found in our air, water, food, and soil. Mercury is found in dental amalgams.

- **Pesticides and herbicides** are ubiquitous in our food supply, even some organic food. Glyphosate is applied to crops worldwide at the rate of five billion pounds per year.

- **Polycyclic aromatic hydrocarbons**, which are products of fossil fuel combustion, especially petrochemicals, are found in polluted air.

- **Bisphenol A (BPA) and phthalates** are chemicals used to make many plastics and resins, including water bottles and food storage containers.

- **Dioxins and dioxin-like chemicals such as polychlorinated biphenyls (PCBs)** are industrial chemicals that are found in contaminated water, soil, and food.

- **Heterocyclic amines** are chemicals that form when food is cooked at high temperatures, especially via grilling or broiling.

One of the primary benefits from any type of fasting is weight loss. As excess weight is a contributing factor to nearly every chronic disease, this is good news. But it does come with a downside: When the weight you lose is in the form of fat, it will typically release the toxins that have been stored in your fat into your bloodstream, exposing you to a flood of toxins. This is a peril your ancestors before the 19th century never faced when they invariably were required to fast, because their bodies hadn't been forced to store these kinds of chemicals.

The U.S. Environmental Protection Agency (EPA)'s National Human Monitoring Program (NHMP), established by the U.S. Public Health Service in 1967, assessed human exposure to toxic substances. Its primary component was the National Human Adipose Tissue Survey (NHATS), performed annually from 1970 to 1989 to collect and chemically analyze human fat specimens for the presence of toxic chemicals. The report clearly documents the extensive amount of chemical exposure occurring in the U.S. population. Interestingly, the last analysis done in 1986 showed significant increases in measured levels of toxins.[2] Additionally, the older the person was, the more likely it was they had acquired more chemical exposures.[3] This is precisely what you would predict. If you are interested, you can download the report at no charge at http://bit.ly/EPA_Analysis.

It is interesting to note that the NHATS data is nearly 40 years old now and it is the most recent analysis we have. You can be certain that the situation has radically worsened since then. One of the problems with fasting in the 21st century is that the world has been inundated with harmful chemicals. More than 85,000 have been introduced to the environment and the food supply in just the past 40 years.

One of the most pernicious and ubiquitous of these chemicals is glyphosate, an herbicide found in Roundup—the most heavily used agricultural chemical of all time, with 1.8 million tons of the stuff used in America alone, and 9.4 million tons used worldwide between 1974 and 2016, according to a study published in the journal *Environmental Sciences Europe*.[4] I should note that although glyphosate was first used in 1974, it wasn't widely used until well after the NHAT studies, which is why it wasn't identified.

The good news is that your body has a built-in protective mechanism that has helped our species survive this growing chemical exposure. The strategy is to store toxic chemicals in your fat to keep them out of your bloodstream where they could harm your body. The bad news is that when you change your diet to go from burning carbs to burning fat, and then you fast on top of it, when your body converts your existing fat stores for energy it will release not only the energy stored in them but also the toxic chemicals that are stored there.

I'll go into further detail on the toxins released during fasting in Chapter 6—please refer to that chapter before attempting any of the fasts I outline here. Also be sure to read the list of contra-indications for fasting in Chapter 5.

INTERMITTENT FASTING: A DEEPER LOOK

There are many different types of intermittent fasting but they all involve regularly switching between eating and not eating—typically for greater than 14 hours in one day. Intermittent fasting is an episodic approach to fasting, and you can implement it a couple of days a month, a couple of days a week, every other day, or even daily, which is what I recommend for most people. It is the first step in the KetoFast program.

Intermittent fasting is rapidly gaining in popularity because it is a profoundly effective strategy that has a broad range of benefits, including weight loss, and radically reducing or eliminating insulin resistance, which is a foundational cause of most chronic degenerative diseases. There is no shortage of information available regarding intermittent fasting and its purported health benefits. In fact, as recently as late 2018, an Internet search using the terms "diet fasting intermittent alternate day" yielded more than 500,000 results—some more useful than others, of course.

While intermittent fasting is not as potent as longer-term fasting, it nevertheless will boost autophagy and mitophagy—your body's natural cleansing processes that are necessary for optimal cellular renewal and function. It also triggers the generation of stem cells and of new mitochondria. There's even evidence to suggest intermittent fasting can help prevent or even help reverse dementia, as it helps your body clean out toxic debris.

Because intermittent fasting lowers insulin resistance, it also increases other important hormones, including growth hormone (known as "the fitness hormone"), which is important for muscle development and general vitality. Just as with cyclical ketosis, most of the rejuvenating and regenerating benefits of intermittent fasting occur during the refeeding phase, not the fasting phase.

THREE BASIC TYPES OF INTERMITTENT FASTING

There are many ways to fast intermittently, and the following are three of the most popular options. Please understand that it is my clinical opinion and strong recommendation that the ideal options for most people are Peak Fasting and KetoFasting, and these alternate methods are simply mentioned to let you know what others have been doing in this area.

- Peak Fasting or Time-Restricted Eating
- KetoFasting or cyclical partial fasting
- Alternate-Day Fasting

Peak Fasting or Time-Restricted Eating (TRE)

Peak Fasting (TRE) is a subset of intermittent fasting and is the practice of limiting your food intake to a certain window of time each day. Peak Fasting gives your body more time to effectively digest what you are eating and to eliminate waste. Many biological repair processes take place when your body is in the "rest," not the "digest," mode, which is one reason why grazing from the time you wake until the time you sleep is a bad strategy.

Restricting your daily eating to a specific window is one intervention that I believe most everyone could implement to experience important health improvements, even if it's the only dietary change you make. For example, if you skip breakfast and make lunch your first meal, your food intake would be between 11 A.M. and 7 P.M. If breakfast suits you better, then your window could be between 8 A.M. and 4 P.M.

The key is to eat only two meals, and to ensure that your last meal ends at least three hours before bedtime. When you eat three or more meals a day, you rarely, if ever, empty your glycogen stores. It takes about 8 to 12 hours to burn most of the sugar stored in your liver as glycogen. Peak Fasting will dramatically improve the way your body processes food for fuel.

Peak Fasting is your first step prior to KetoFasting, as it will help your body regain the ability to burn fat for fuel and become metabolically flexible. You engage in the process as long as it takes for your body to create ketones. Ketones can be measured easily from your urine, blood, or even your breath.

Once your body is able to create ketones regularly, you can begin to incorporate additional carbs and protein into your diet several days a week, ideally on days when you are exercising vigorously or strength training. Another term for this is cyclical ketosis. Some advocate continuous ketosis, but I believe that will result in complications for most people. Nature follows cycles, and so should your food intake. After you have regained metabolic flexibility, you need variation in your diet, and cyclical ketosis achieves this in spades. You can continue on cyclical ketosis indefinitely or, even better, progress to KetoFasting, which will help your body repair and regenerate while removing toxins that you have accumulated from living in the 21st century.

KetoFasting—a Type of Partial Fasting

One of the best ways for the average person to improve their health is with a partial metabolically supported fast—or what I call KetoFasting. I believe KetoFasting delivers the best possible mixture of fasting benefits and compliance, especially when it is incorporated into a cyclical ketogenic diet (as I will explain how to do in Chapter 8). It is also a key strategy for minimizing the potential of exposure to toxins that are liberated from your fat stores when you fast.

When you are metabolically flexible (able to burn fat for fuel) and you engage in this method, your body will mobilize the toxins from your fat cells. When KetoFasting, you eat a limited number of nutrient-dense foods—particularly foods that contain phytonutrients—that support detoxification during your partial fast, helping your body to effectively metabolize and eliminate these toxins. Once the toxins are processed and liberated—and sweated out with the assistance of a sauna, or excreted into your bile—it will be important to bind the toxins so that they can be eliminated and not reabsorbed. There are a wide variety of safe and inexpensive binding agents that can help you achieve this.

I strongly recommend that anyone who is starting a fasting regimen consider a strategy that creates the benefits of fasting, while also mitigating the potential downsides—primarily, the risk for toxic overload. You may have heard of many horror stories or side effects of those who have tried to fast. Maybe you have even tried fasting yourself and had a negative experience. It is my strong belief that these negative side effects are largely due to improperly supported detoxification systems: your body is simply unable to properly process the liberated toxins released when stored fat is burned as fuel.

Regardless, there are other important reasons to engage in Keto-Fasting rather than attempting a water-only fast. A major reason to undertake a supported fast is that when your body undergoes lipolysis—or fat burning—the phytonutrients in the foods that you eat on your fasting days, if chosen carefully, will actually help your body process and metabolize toxins so you can effectively eliminate them from your body and minimize or avoid any negative side effects.

Alternate-Day Fasting

In this version of intermittent fasting, you alternate between eating normally one day and restricting your intake to one meal of about 500 calories or less for the next. This method has been popularized by Krista Varady, Ph.D., author of *The Every-Other-Day Diet.*

A positive aspect of alternate-day fasting is that it provides a nice rhythm that makes it relatively easy to adapt to—just as you are getting hungry, it is time to break your fast. You could even fast from dinnertime to dinnertime, achieving 24 hours of fasting while still eating one meal each day.

Varady's clinical trial of alternate-day fasting found that only 10 percent of people couldn't stick to the program while about 90 percent of participants were able to follow the schedule for 16 weeks.[5] People in the fasting group saw significant reductions in weight, body-fat mass, triglycerols, C-reactive protein (a marker of inflammation), and the hunger hormone leptin.

This is likely a beneficial method to counteract obesity, as it will drop weight quickly. But it is simply too much fasting, which, as we've covered, can create a toxic environment in your body if you don't approach it carefully. For that reason, I believe that alternate-day fasting is not a suitable long-term solution. One rodent study found that animals kept on an alternate-day fasting program long term experienced diminished alternate diastolic reserve in the heart,[6] and this makes sense to me. This kind of fasting, long term, is likely to do more harm than good.

IMPLEMENTING KETOFASTING

If you are like most people and have lost your metabolic flexibility—which is to say, you are currently unable to burn fat for fuel and rely primarily on carbs for fuel—this will be challenging. You may experience hunger either at night or in the morning, and you may notice your energy dipping; this is because your body is sending hunger signals in an attempt to get you to provide more glucose to use for fuel and your energy will crash as your glycogen stores run out.

The good news is that for most people, this uncomfortable transition period only lasts a few weeks, and there are several tips that can radically improve your discomfort during this time.

Once you can burn fat for fuel, these symptoms will improve dramatically. But until you become metabolically flexible, if you experience hunger or low energy, drinking a glass of water or sipping a cup of bone broth can help tide you over. You can also add a teaspoon or two of coconut oil or ghee to your morning coffee or tea, which will help address those hunger pangs without raising your blood sugar. Just make sure that the coconut oil you buy has the words "hexane-free" and "chemical-free" on the label, as some brands use hexane—a neurotoxin—and other harmful chemicals to extract more oil from the coconuts. You don't want to expose yourself to additional toxins, especially when you are embarking on a program to eliminate fat-stored toxins from the body.

Remember, once you have become fat-adapted, you will find it easy to go 18 hours or even longer without food because your hunger will recede and your energy will remain steady as you will always have plenty of access to fat (from the fat cells in your own body) to burn for fuel. The longer you are fat-adapted, the easier it will be to go longer and longer periods of time during each day without eating.

Once you have made a 12-hour eating window a normal part of your life, which is typically a few weeks for most, begin experimenting with reducing the time frame in which you eat to 11, 10, and eventually down to 6 to 8 hours. By doing so, you will give your body access to greater periods of repair and restoration.

When you nudge your non-eating window into the realm of only 16 to 18 hours a day, you will allow your body sufficient downtime to drain your glycogen stores—a necessary precursor to shifting into burning fat for fuel and having your liver pump out ketones.

If you would like some technological assistance in this effort, Dr. Satchin Panda of the Salk Institute has developed an app called myCircadianClock. It will help you log what you eat and set a daily eating window target, with reminders to help you.

Remember, no matter how long your daily window of fasting is, the key is to ensure that you eat your last meal at least three hours before bedtime. For this reason, if you need to skip a meal in order to meet your daily fasting goal, it might make sense to skip dinner instead, or eat early, instead of skipping breakfast. I realize that for most people, especially those with families and those who work until well into the evening, this is challenging.

Time with family and friends is an essential component of health and I am not suggesting you abandon that. However, consider altering the experience slightly. Spend the mealtime with your family or friends but adjust your own food. You could drink a cup of tea or a glass of carbonated water instead of eating and still engage in your relationships. You might also choose to shrink your portion size significantly, or if you're dining out, order a small appetizer or side salad rather than a full entrée.

I know some of you with obsessive-compulsive tendencies (I include myself in this group) may think that if restricting your eating to only a six- to eight-hour window is good, then a four- or even a two-hour window would be even better. I would rather see you put your efforts into KetoFasting, which involves adopting a cyclical ketogenic diet that's eaten during only a moderately compressed eating window, and then periodically giving yourself the experience of a longer fast—all of which will help you reap more of the benefits of fasting in a very doable way. I'll explain exactly how to do this in Chapter 8.

First, though, we'll address a common question: Is it *safe* to fast? I know that many people worry about this, thinking that fasting can be dangerous and may lead to starvation, wasting away, or even death. So to remove any mental barriers of this kind that may be keeping you from embracing a regular fast, in the next chapter we'll take a close look at the research on whether fasting is safe.

SUMMARY

- Intermittent fasting, also known as time-restricted eating, involves fasting for at least 14 to 16 hours every day and eating all of your meals within 6 to 8 consecutive hours.

- Partial fasting consists of eating a very limited number of calories in order to encourage a physiological state of fasting.

- Water fasting requires that only water is consumed; it is best performed under medical supervision.

- One danger of water fasting is that it can liberate large amounts of toxins stored in your fat cells that will not be detoxified properly and therefore will likely contribute to toxin resorption and many side effects.

- KetoFasting is a 300- to 600-calorie, nutrient-dense partial fast, typically performed once or twice a week following a 16- to 18-hour intermittent fast.

- For maximum benefits, one should adopt a cyclical ketogenic diet prior to starting KetoFasting to become metabolically flexible and able to burn fat for fuel and minimize hunger or other side effects during the very low-calorie partial-fast days.

CHAPTER 5

IS FASTING SAFE?

With the conventional nutritional wisdom suggesting you should eat three meals a day, plus two small snacks, the mere mention that you are thinking of abstaining from food for a day can be perceived as crazy by well-meaning friends, family members, and even medical professionals. They may even tell you it's outright dangerous.

Is there any merit to the perception that therapeutic fasting is unsafe?

One of the biggest worries about going extended periods without food is that your body will start cannibalizing itself as a result of starvation and that your muscles will wither away, your health will decline, and if you keep going long enough, you will die prematurely as a result of this foolish endeavor.

Much of this belief stems from a period when extreme forms of water fasting were used to treat obesity. During this time there were several deaths reported—likely the result of unintentionally harmful fasting practices.

Yet the majority of us have enough reserves of body fat to safely undergo a water fast for at least 40 days before we worsen our health and go into starvation mode. How long any individual can safely fast will vary according to their fat and muscle percentages, nutrient reserves, and overall state of health. In the simplest terms, the more body fat you have, the longer you will be able to fast (barring any health contraindications, which are covered later in this chapter). It is only when your fat stores have been exhausted that your body turns to consuming your muscles and soft tissues, such as your organs. If this is left unchecked, it will ultimately progress to death. But again, this would only happen after your fat stores were completely exhausted. Since most people have substantial fat stores, they can live about 40 days without food.

That being said, please understand that I do *not* recommend that you attempt a water fast of any duration, much less 40 days, without qualified professional supervision, as there are many complications that can result. It is far safer, healthier, and more comfortable to use the KetoFast partial-fasting protocol where you consume 300 to 600 calories (based on your lean body weight) of foods that will support your detoxification process, which will be activated once you liberate fat-soluble toxins from your fat cells.

It is my hope that the information here will convince you that careful, intentional fasting is perfectly safe.

SIDE EFFECTS AND BENEFITS OF FASTING

The negative side effects one may experience from fasting will vary from person to person. In many cases, they are caused by fat-soluble toxins that get released into your bloodstream once fats are being burned for fuel. The most typical symptoms include headaches, insomnia, nausea, back pain, indigestion, fatigue, skin irritations, body odor, aching limbs, palpitations, mucous discharge, and visual and hearing disturbances. Electrolyte imbalance is by far the most serious side effect of fasting.

These symptoms are generally transient, although for some people, more significant complications can occur, in which case the fast must be terminated. Examples of serious complications include sudden drop in blood pressure; delirium; prolonged hypothermia; rapid, slow, or irregular pulse; extreme weakness;

vomiting and diarrhea leading to dehydration; kidney problems; gout; emotional distress; and significant electrolyte imbalance.

Despite these unpleasant side effects, fasting—even extended water fasting (when done under medical supervision)—is increasingly recognized as a safe and highly effective therapy for a wide number of diseases, including hypertension, appendicitis, cardiovascular disease, follicular lymphoma, and as a powerful adjunct to chemotherapy.

The reason why fasting is so effective in conjunction with chemotherapy is that cancer cells rely primarily on burning sugar through glycolysis. When you fast, you limit glucose availability, which is the cancer cells' primary fuel, yet you still have plenty of oxygen available to metabolize nutrients via the Krebs cycle, a far more effective method of energy production.

But cancer cells are intelligent and have another strategy for creating energy by burning an amino acid called glutamine, which it can scavenge from muscles. Some astute researchers, such as Dr. Thomas Seyfried, are using glutamine inhibitors to make cancer cells even more energy deprived and susceptible to chemotherapy. One common glutamine inhibitor is epigallocatechin-3-gallate (EGCG) from green tea at around 400 milligrams.[1]

If you have any friends or relatives who are considering chemotherapy for treating cancer, it is highly recommended that they integrate water fasting the day before and the day of chemotherapy, as it will not only radically decrease the side effects of the chemo but will likely increase the chemo's effectiveness. Ideally, water fasting should be preceded by a KetoFasting regimen to increase metabolic flexibility prior to the water fast.

Many cancer patients have cancer cachexia and are underweight, so again this strategy should only be implemented with the assistance of a knowledgeable health-care professional.

ABSOLUTE AND RELATIVE
CONTRAINDICATIONS FOR KETOFASTING

Most people could safely benefit from intermittent fasting (time-restricted eating) as you are not necessarily restricting calorie intake. However, if you are going to engage in the KetoFast protocol (outlined in Chapter 8), it would be best to avoid Keto-Fasting until the following conditions have improved or resolved.

Absolute Contraindications

- **Underweight.** Refrain from any type of fasting if you have a body mass index (BMI) of 18.5 or less.

- **Malnourished.** You need to put your focus on eating healthier, more nutritious food before you can safely do any kind of fast. I would also caution you to avoid fasting if you struggle with an eating disorder such as anorexia, even if you are not clinically underweight.

- **Pregnancy and breastfeeding.** Pregnant and breast-feeding women put their baby's healthy growth and development at risk when fasting because a consistent flow of nutrients must be shared continually with the baby to ensure his or her well-being.

Relative Contraindications

It's important to exercise caution with fasting if any of the following conditions apply to you, unless you are carefully supervised by a qualified health-care professional.

- **Age.** Children should not fast for more than 24 hours because they need nutrients for continued growth; if your child is obese and has a serious condition like autism, there may be benefit from KetoFasting under the guidance of a qualified health-care professional.

- **Certain medications.** If you take medication and it must be taken with food to achieve the proper effect, you will need to use caution when fasting. Medications such as aspirin and metformin, as well as any other drugs that may cause stomach ulcers or stomach upset, need to be considered.

   Risks are especially high if you're taking any medications, especially for diabetes or hypertension. If you take the same dose of medication while you are fasting, you run the risk of your blood sugar or blood pressure dropping too low. In these circumstances you will need to find a qualified health-care practitioner to guide you through the process of adjusting your dosages to suit your KetoFast plan.

- **High uric acid or a tendency toward gout.** Fasting tends to increase your uric acid level because your kidneys increase their reabsorption of uric acid when you don't eat. Most people will not experience a problem with this, but if you have gout it would be wise to consult with a knowledgeable health-care professional.

SUMMARY

- Despite popular misconceptions, the average human has enough fat stores to last for approximately 40 days without food.

- Fasting does have some common side effects, including headaches, insomnia, nausea, back pain, indigestion, fatigue, skin irritations, body odor, aching limbs, palpitations, mucous discharge, and visual and hearing disturbances. Generally these are short-lived and are the result of toxins being liberated from your fat cells.

- More serious side effects, which indicate that you should stop your fasting practice, are sudden drop in blood pressure; delirium; prolonged hypothermia; rapid, slow, or irregular pulse; extreme weakness; vomiting and diarrhea leading to dehydration; kidney problems; gout; emotional distress; and significant electrolyte imbalance.

- Water fasting is believed to be helpful during cancer treatment, particularly on the day before and day of chemotherapy treatment.

- If you are underweight, malnourished, pregnant, or breastfeeding, you should not undergo any kind of fasting treatment.

- Children, those who are on regular medications, and those who have a tendency toward gout should fast only with medical supervision.

CHAPTER 6

THE DARK SIDE OF FASTING

As beneficial as fasting can be, if not done properly it has one potentially serious downside. As discussed, when you are in a fasted state and your body begins to burn your fat stores, it releases the toxins that have been stored in your fat tissue. If your detoxification pathways are not optimally supported, this can wreak havoc on your body. This is a peril your ancestors before the 19th century never faced when they were required to fast, because the environment simply wasn't contaminated to the extent that it is today.

The good news is that your body has ancient pre-programmed protective mechanisms that have helped our species survive toxic exposures. Your body stores these toxic chemicals in your fat to keep them out of your bloodstream where they could harm your body. The bad news is that when you fast and your body burns your existing fat stores for fuel (a process called lipolysis), it will release not only the energy, but also the toxic chemicals that are stored there as well.

THE PREVALENCE OF TOXIC CHEMICALS

Today, fat-soluble toxins are widespread throughout the environment. Nearly every activity leaves behind some kind of waste. Cars, trucks, and buses emit toxic exhaust fumes while in operation. Industrial and manufacturing processes create solid and hazardous waste material that leaches chemicals into our air, soil, and water supply. The spraying of our food with millions of tons of herbicides and pesticides also contributes to this exposure. Over five million pounds of glyphosate alone are sprayed annually.

Many of these toxic compounds are resistant to degradation and persist in the environment and in our food for long periods of time. As a result, chemical toxin levels in humans have skyrocketed and are now found in people across the globe.[1, 2, 3] Worse yet, there are many reasons to consider these compounds a threat to human health.[4, 5] Because of the ubiquitous contamination of foods with toxic materials, a vast majority of the U.S. population—up to 99.9 percent, depending on the particular toxin—have been found to have measurable levels of various chemical toxins,[6] including heavy metals such as arsenic, cadmium, and lead.[7] The artificial sweetener sucralose has also recently been found to accumulate in the fat tissues of rats[8]—something I predicted in my 2008 book *Sweet Deception*.

The newest term for most of these fat-soluble toxins is persistent organic pollutants (POPs).[9] POPs are present in our water, food, and air.[10] They usually come from various agricultural and industrial activities such as overuse of pesticides and synthesis of fertilizers. POPs are characterized by their ability to persist in the environment, their high fat-solubility, and their bioaccumulation in the food chain.[11]

The toxicity of many of these compounds has been studied extensively. Higher exposure to POPs has been associated with an increase in reactive oxygen species (ROS) that can lead to cell inflammation[12, 13] and increased oxidative stress.[14] Exposure to POPs can also alter metabolic mechanisms, resulting in insulin resistance,[15] obesity,[16] dyslipidemia,[17] and type 2 diabetes.[18]

POPs are also associated with chronic diseases—such as cancer, cardiovascular disease, neurodegenerative disease, and respiratory disease[19, 20]—and, more important, an increase in all-cause mortality.[21]

POPs include many compounds found in organochlorine pesticides such as dieldrin, DDT, and chlordane, along with several industrial chemical products or by-products such as polychlorinated biphenyls (PCBs), flame retardants known as PBDEs, and plasticizers like phthalates and bisphenol A (BPA). Another POP is perfluorooctanoic acid (PFOA), a man-made chemical containing fluoride that is most often found in nonstick coatings for cookware.[22]

PBDEs are mixtures of chemicals used as flame retardants in many consumer products such as upholstery, plastics, and cabinets.[23] Exposure to PBDEs often occurs through ingesting contaminated dust, food, and breastmilk; touching contaminated soil or commercial products; and inhaling contaminated air.[24] Studies suggest that exposure to PBDEs is associated with changes in neurodevelopment.[25, 26]

PCBs include manufactured mixtures of chlorinated compounds used as lubricants and coolants in electrical equipment, as well as in industrial applications such as plasticizers and pigments.[27] The production of PCBs in the U.S. ended in 1979 due to concern about potential health effects.[28] In 2004 many countries eliminated the production and use of PCBs in accordance with the Stockholm Convention.[29] However, because PCBs persist in the environment for many years, exposure is still occurring, and increasing evidence suggests that even low-level exposure to PCBs may have adverse health consequences.[30, 31] The EPA classifies PCBs as probable human carcinogens,[32] although there is still debate about whether exposure increases the risk of mortality in the general population.[33, 34]

Many of the toxins mentioned have been shown to inhibit enzyme activities in the mitochondrial electron transport chain,[35] which is a problem, as this is where most of the energy in your body is produced. There is some good news here: What you eat can affect how harmful POPs are once they are in your body,[36] both positively and negatively. For example, linoleic acid (an omega-6 fatty acid) can increase the toxicity of PCB in vascular endothelial cells, but this effect can be mitigated by vitamin E. Omega-3 essential fats and polyphenols have been shown to reduce many conditions that are associated with the presence of toxins, including tumor formation and growth, liver diseases, and endothelial cell activation.[37]

This modulating effect of certain foods highlights the importance of eating a high-quality, nutrient-dense diet before, after, and even during fasting (in calorically limited amounts) in order to mitigate the potential risk of toxin reexposure. For example, plant-derived flavonoids such as EGCG can decrease oxidative stress and inflammation.[38]

HEAVY METAL TOXICITY AND HEART HEALTH

Stored heavy metals have been associated with heart risks. An analysis published in the *BMJ* (*British Medical Journal*) in 2018 looked at data on about 350,000 people from 37 different countries and found that exposure to commonly found heavy metals such as arsenic (present in pressure-treated wood, electronics, and herbicides[39]), lead (still prevalent in the environment after years of use in gasoline, water pipes, and paint), cadmium (present in many fertilizers), and copper (a by-product of many industries that can build up in soil and drinking water[40]) are associated with an increased incidence of cardiovascular disease and mortality. Sadly, even minimal exposure to these metals showed increased risk.[41]

The good news is that removing heavy metals from your body has been shown to reduce the risk of cardiovascular disease. A clinical study sponsored by the National Institutes of Health and the National Center for Complementary and Integrative Health called TACT (Trial to Assess Chelation Therapy)[42] looked at the effectiveness of chelation—a blood detoxifying therapy popular in the alternative medicine world—and nutritional supplements at reducing cardiovascular events.

This incredibly expensive study—the NIH spent $31.6 million on it—found that chelation therapy, when given in combination with high doses of vitamins, reduced the risk of cardiovascular events by 18 percent, and this lower risk lasted for five years after the end of the study. When patients either received chelation therapy with no supplements or took vitamin supplements but did not get chelation therapy, the risk reduction was much lower than when they were combined. These findings strongly suggest that the presence of heavy metals in your body is dangerous, and you need extra nutrition to support detoxification.

TOXIC EXPOSURE AS A RESULT OF FASTING IN HUMANS

Remember the early 1990s Biosphere 2 experiment, for which eight scientists entered a sealed glass and steel structure that contained its own ecosystem in the Arizona desert and stayed there for nearly two years? Well, their experience validated the concerns of toxin release during fasting. One of the Biosphere 2 participants, Ray Walford, a physician and pioneer of caloric restriction,[43] reported increased levels of organochlorine compounds in individuals who lost weight during the experiment.

More recently, several studies of stored fat-soluble toxins report that loss of body fat results in mobilization of toxins and their redistribution into other tissues and organs.[44, 45, 46] Other studies show that those who underwent bariatric surgery released significant amounts of POPs from fat stores after their subsequent weight loss.[47] Another study showed that those who weighed more and had higher levels of fat stores had significantly more toxins in their system.[48]

WHY MOST ARE UNABLE TO KEEP THE
WEIGHT OFF ONCE THEY LOSE IT

While weight reduction is difficult in and of itself, anyone who has ever lost weight will confirm that it is much harder to keep the weight off once it has been lost than it is to lose it in the first place. In fact, more than 80 percent of people who lose weight relapse to pre-weight-loss levels of body fat. Many experts believe the reason why this happens is because of metabolic, behavioral, neuroendocrine, and autonomic responses designed to maintain body fat, which store fat at a neurologically defined "ideal" level. Collectively known as adaptive thermogenesis, these responses create the ideal situation for weight regain; many experts believe this is the reason both lean and obese individuals attempting to sustain reduced body weight are unsuccessful.[49] While this is the commonly accepted reason why most overweight individuals fail to keep their lost weight off, it may not be the true cause. The root of weight regain may actually be the liberation of toxins that happens during the weight-loss process.

A fascinating study showed that increased POPs in the blood seems to be a major factor affecting adaptive thermogenesis in some obese individuals, even more so than thyroid hormone and leptin levels.[50] It has also been shown that the total body burden of POPs is greater in obese people than in lean individuals because of the larger concentration of POPs in their plasma and fat,[51] so when they lose weight, the concentration of POPs in their blood increases.[52, 53] Once the POPs are shifted into your blood from the fat stores (where you have been protected from them) they are more able to exert their adverse effects on metabolism.

The increase in POP concentration caused by weight loss has been shown to be an independent predictor of a decrease in plasma thyroid hormone levels,[54] resting metabolic rate, and skeletal muscle oxidative enzyme activity.[55] Considering that POPs are also known to alter the function of your mitochondria,[56] it is likely that the increase in plasma POPs is a factor in regaining weight after losing it.[57, 58]

FASTING ANIMAL STUDIES CONFIRMING
FAT-STORED TOXINS

Even as early as 1962, it was shown that partial fasting resulted in the mobilization of fat-soluble toxins like DDT from the fat deposits of rats who were fed nontoxic levels of DDT.[59]

Many marine mammals (seals in particular) go through extensive periods of fasting during reproduction, migration, molting, and post-weaning. During such periods, they burn their blubber fat reserves and, as a result, liberate PCBs and other fat-soluble chemicals into their blood.[60, 61, 62] Dramatically higher levels of PCBs have been found in the blood of thin adult harp seals—sampled during the molt, when body condition is poor—than in fat adult harp seals—sampled during the breeding season.[63]

Northern elephant seals are characterized by extended periods of fasting during which they rely entirely on their own body fat reserves. This has been documented to free toxic fat-soluble pollutants like PCBs into their blood circulation.[64, 65]

Researchers have shown that an adequate diet aiming at weight loss induced a significant increase in blood levels of POPs,[66] and, more important, significantly decreased the ability of muscles to burn fat for fuel.[67] Another study showed that fat-soluble toxins were increased in the brains and kidneys of mice when body fat was lost.[68]

HOW YOUR BODY DETOXES
HARMFUL SUBSTANCES

When you are exposed to these pernicious 20th- and 21st-century toxins, your body has evolved brilliant protective mechanisms that cause those toxins to get locked away in your fat cells where they cause limited damage to your body. However, once you burn the fat in the cells where these toxins are stored, they are released back into your body.

So what to do? If you are healthy, this is typically not a problem as you have generalized detoxification mechanisms located in your liver that convert fat-soluble toxins to water-soluble toxins so your body can eliminate them in your sweat, urine, or stool.

The Four Stages of Detoxification

Unfortunately, conventional chelation therapy is expensive, frequently not covered by insurance, and inconvenient. Alternatively and thankfully, KetoFasting is an effective way to liberate and eliminate these toxins, plus it is inexpensive, convenient, and flexible. That being said, it is important to understand how to support your body's detoxification process to maximize the benefits of KetoFasting.

Ridding your body of toxins follows four distinct stages. If there are hiccups in any of the stages, liberated toxins will not be expelled by your body, but instead may be reabsorbed where they will contribute to cellular damage.

- **Phase Zero:** The toxin enters the cell, still in its fat-soluble state. This can happen either through environmental exposure or as the result of lipolysis.

- **Phase One:** A hydroxyl group is added to the toxin, making it water-soluble (and therefore able to be excreted). Although this is a vital part of the process that ultimately leads to removing the toxin from your body, in this state the toxin is still highly reactive and dangerous. You want to be able to move it along through the next two phases as quickly as possible.

- **Phase Two:** In a process called conjugation, something gets added to the toxin that makes it much less volatile and destructive: either a methyl group, a sulphur group, an acetyl group, or an amino acid such as glycine or glutathione. This added structure quiets the toxin and makes it far less reactive and damaging while it is in the process of being eliminated by your body.

- **Phase Three.** This is the crucial part, when the toxin leaves the cell and moves along the path to being excreted, either through your sweat, urine, or stool.

It's important during phase one and two to consume enough of the types of nutrients that support your detoxification pathways, allowing your body to safely convert the toxins to a water-soluble form that your body can eliminate easily.

By following a cyclical ketogenic diet on the days when you are not KetoFasting, and eating plenty of low-net-carb vegetables such as broccoli, cauliflower, and cabbage, you will provide you liver with the nutrients it needs to be able to process these freed toxins.

Next you will want to facilitate the elimination of these toxins from your body by doing things that encourage sweating, such as using a near-infrared (NIR) sauna, and drinking plenty of water to encourage urination.

Additionally, using binders to capture the toxins that are excreted by your liver into your stool will help to eliminate them rather than allowing them to be reabsorbed. Fiber is an important binder that enhances toxin excretion from your bowels. Some of the more popular, safe, and inexpensive binders that you can take include activated charcoal, chlorella, chitosan, and modified citrus pectin. (See Chapter 8 for more information on each of these.)

The trouble is, most people have not been following a clean, nutrient-dense diet and exercising regularly, and as a result are generally not very healthy. If you are deficient in any of the nutrients that support detoxification, the process will be impaired and you will likely experience symptoms during KetoFasting. More important, your body will not be able to effectively eliminate and remove the toxins from your system. This is why, even though I am a proponent of medically supervised water fasting for very serious conditions, I believe that it is far wiser for most people to take the more conservative and slower approach of KetoFasting, because it is carefully designed to support your body in its quest to effectively eliminate toxins.

KetoFasting will provide you with 300 to 600 calories of nutrient-dense foods that are full of phytonutrients that will support detoxification as well as your ability to convert liberated fat-soluble toxins into water-soluble toxins that can be eliminated from your body.

Difference Between Active and Passive Sweating

While almost of us sweat when we exercise intensely, active sweating is not as effective for toxin elimination as passive sweating.

Again, while you certainly can sweat up a storm with exercise, if you're working on detoxifying heavy metals and other pernicious toxins from your body, passive sweating is far more effective than active sweating. Active sweating is caused by physical exertion such as during exercise. Research has shown that the toxin concentration in sweat during exercise is actually quite low. Perhaps even more important, when you are KetoFasting, you really don't want to engage in vigorous exercise as this will impair your body's ability to maximize the benefits of partial fasting.

Sweat samples taken during sauna bathing, on the other hand—i.e., during passive sweating—reveal that high amounts of toxins are being released in the sweat. The reason for this has to do with sympathetic versus parasympathetic nervous system activation. Your autonomic nervous system has two states, commonly referred to as "fight or flight" and "rest and digest."

When you're exercising vigorously enough to start sweating, your body is allocating energy toward your muscles, lungs, and heart. This is fight-or-flight time. During passive sweating, however, your body is heated from the outside rather than from within, a much more restful state. Since you're not exerting yourself in any way, your body is able to use the energy generated from the incandescent heat lamps to heal and repair itself, as it decides that this is a good time to release toxins through your sweat.

When you are not physically exerting yourself, the sympathetic nervous system quiets down and your parasympathetic nervous (PNS) system comes online. The PNS rules the rest and repair functions of your body, and that includes detoxification.

SAUNA THERAPY

While it is certainly possible to do KetoFasting without access to a sauna, it is not ideal; in fact, you will experience fewer benefits. Remember, one of the primary benefits of KetoFasting is to help you eliminate toxins, and it is very difficult to do this optimally without access to a sauna. If at all possible, it should be in your home so it is convenient and you will use it.

The Differences Between Near- and Far-IR Saunas

The vast majority of infrared saunas are far IR. While these certainly have many benefits, they also have many drawbacks. The difference between far and near IR is the wavelength of the light. Near-infrared light is just beyond the light spectrum of visible red light; it starts around 700 nanometers and goes up to 1,400 nanometers. Mid-infrared ranges from 1,400 to 3,000 nanometers, and far infrared is from 3,000 to 100,000 nanometers.

It is important to understand these frequencies as they have significant biological consequences. Near IR can penetrate into your body up to 100 millimeters (3.9 inches), while far IR only penetrates a few millimeters, or a tiny fraction of an inch. Even though far IR has more energy than near IR, water in your body absorbs the radiation from far IR before it can penetrate effectively into your tissues.

Let me explain. Water absorbs different wavelengths to different degrees. Water starts absorbing the energy at about 980 nanometers—right in the middle of the near-IR spectrum. But it's a continuum, so once you get out of near IR, at about 1,400 or 1,500 nanometers, the water is absorbing nearly all the wavelengths and virtually none of the infrared is entering your body.

Once you get out to mid IR, and certainly when you get to far IR wavelengths, they're 100 percent absorbed by water. Many people are unaware of this, but far-IR wavelengths, for that reason, do not penetrate biological tissue or your body very deeply. This means that far-IR saunas are essentially surface-heating you, and heating you in a conductive fashion. With near-IR wavelengths, you get radiant, penetrating heat. This is a much more efficient way to heat biological tissues.

You can observe a similar effect when you are outside on a sunny summer day and feel the heat of the sun on your skin. When a cloud passes over, the warmth disappears instantly. Did you ever wonder why? It is because clouds are loaded with water. They absorb the far infrared and it never reaches your skin, so you don't heat up.

Near IR Activates Your Body's Innate Capacity for Healing

Most people who have studied natural approaches to health—whether formally or informally—understand how important regular sunlight exposure is to our health. And nearly everyone understands that exposure to sunlight creates vitamin D in your skin (far better than swallowing vitamin D capsules). It is exposure to ultraviolet B (UVB) wavelengths that causes your body to make vitamin D.

Traditionally, the benefit of sun exposure is thought to be almost universally due to the benefit of UVB radiation. You might be surprised to learn that UVB in sunlight is less than one-half of one percent of the sunlight spectrum. What most overlook is the effect of near IR and its impact on our biology. This is important, as 40 percent of sunlight—yes, 40 percent, or nearly 100 times more than UVB—is in the near-IR spectrum, which strongly supports the idea that this is an important frequency to be exposed to.

Photobiomodulation (PBM) is the term used to describe light's beneficial effects in your body. Interestingly, near IR has a number of wavelengths that provide PBM effects, including helping your mitochondria become more efficient in producing energy and reducing the production of reactive oxygen species (ROS) and oxidative stresses that can contribute to inflammation.

In addition to activating your mitochondria, near IR helps to structure the water in your body and provide it with energy that can be used in a variety of ways. (Structured water is a more ordered form of water that acts as a vehicle to activate, improve, and optimize biological systems.)

Far-IR frequencies do not appear to have any PBM impacts on your mitochondria. In addition to activating your mitochondria, near IR and red light that is also present in heat lamp bulbs helps to structure the water in your body and provide it with energy that can be used in a variety of different ways. So now you understand that sunlight exposure is doing more than heating your body or promoting vitamin D production. It actually activates an entire healing system. Since you have mitochondria in every cell of your body, with the exception of red blood cells, it's a core restorative healing system.

Far-IR Saunas Often Misrepresent Their Benefits

In contrast, far-IR frequencies do not appear to have any PBM impacts on your mitochondria. Remember, far-IR saunas are NOT providing radiant heat; instead, they heat your body by conduction, which is why you have to heat them up to a relatively high temperature before you go in or you simply won't sweat. They do heat your body, but at a very superficial level, reaching only a few millimeters into your tissues.

Two other common problems with far-IR saunas are that they claim to be "full-spectrum," when in fact they emit virtually no near IR, and they emit high levels of electromagnetic fields (EMFs), even if claiming to be low- or no-EMF emitting.

I've measured many low-EMF, far-IR saunas, and while there were many with very low *magnetic* fields (the "M" in EMF), they virtually all emitted high amounts of *electric* fields (the "E" in EMF), and many had extraordinarily high and dangerous electric fields.

There are many so-called full-spectrum far-IR saunas now that have far-IR emitters for heat, but they've added in near-IR emitters in one of two ways. One way is to use LEDs. You can make digital LEDs now that emit only a few monochromatic near-IR wavelengths and not the full range of more than 700 frequencies in the near-IR spectrum. But it still doesn't have the same natural spectral power curve shape as an incandescent bulb (or sunlight).

There are also some saunas that use low-energy near-IR emitters that are basically heating elements that are hotter than the far IRs. They do emit a small amount of near IR, but it's at a very low power level (what is termed *irradiance* in light-therapy) and has very little biological impact.

The Benefits of Incandescent Near-IR Heating

The incandescent light bulb is the most efficient way to heat your sauna—and thus, your body—because it is almost exclusively full-spectrum near IR. While incandescent light bulbs use far more energy than LED bulbs, the heating they provide actually has profound therapeutic benefits. Farmers have long used incandescent light bulbs to incubate animal life and keep livestock warm, for example. Incandescent light bulbs can also be used for incandescent sauna therapy.

Sadly, the U.S. and most of Europe has shifted to LEDs and fluorescents to reduce energy consumption. Doing so has removed many of the healing wavelengths of light for the sake of energy efficiency, but with very detrimental consequences to your health. It's not just about detox.

There are so many aspects of incandescent sauna therapy that are beneficial. Essentially, what you're doing with near-IR sauna therapy is stimulating your mitochondria to release nitric oxide (NO) from one of the proteins in the electron transport chain in the mitochondria, which stimulates adenosine triphosphate (ATP) production, in addition to structuring the water in your cells. Together, your mitochondria, NO, and ATP work in concert to promote healing effects such as DNA repair and cellular regeneration.

Therapeutic Dosing

Even with light therapy, you don't want excessive exposure. Just like you can't be in the sun for an unlimited amount of time, you don't want to be in the sauna for eight hours. A sauna heat-shocks your body, promoting detox and other beneficial cellular responses—but you don't want to stay shocked for too long. A 20- to 30-minute near-IR sauna session delivers the appropriate amount of energy (around 36 to 54 joules at a distance of 1½ to 2 feet from the bulbs).

Accessing Your Own Incandescent Sauna

There are a number of companies that produce heat-lamp near-IR saunas. SaunaSpace is one of the best, as it has a No-EMF version that not only has no electric and magnetic fields but also shields against radiofrequency waves from cellphones and Wi-Fi, creating an ideal parasympathetic detox environment. However, they are expensive.

The least-expensive approach would be to build your own near-IR sauna with Teflon-free heat lamps. Instructions can be found in Dr. Lawrence Wilson's book *Sauna Therapy for Detoxification and Healing*, available on Amazon. This type of sauna was used in Dr. John Harvey Kellogg's sanitariums and spas in the early 1900s. The core of the sauna is four 250-watt Philips incandescent bulbs, which can be purchased for less than $40. You just want to make sure that there is no Teflon on the bulb to prevent vaporizing fluoride and breathing it in. Although far less expensive, this approach does have some serious disadvantages and requires some care and attention. First, all materials need to be toxin-free and hypoallergenic. Natural materials are best and off-gassing plastics should be avoided.

Second, the heat lamp bulbs get very hot. You don't want to touch the surface of an incandescent bulb, for you can burn yourself. You need professional protection from that, and a hardware cloth or some flexible wire is typically not sufficient and will expose you to burn damage.

The third alternative and midtier cost would be a hybrid approach. You can purchase the fixtures and bulb protectors from companies that sell the full near-IR saunas, but use your own enclosure. The fixtures are typically diamond-shaped with one bulb on the top and bottom and two bulbs in the middle.

The heating you want occurs as a result of the light shining onto your body, so you don't really need a sauna tent. All you really need is the air around you to be above body temperature; above 100 degrees Fahrenheit, which happens very quickly once you turn the bulbs on. You can hang the heat-lamp-bulb fixture in your shower or even a dedicated closet or small room.

But be careful if using a small room. If surrounding materials like paint or finished wood or carpet have petrochemicals in them, undesirable toxic off-gassing can occur. Also, since the heating is directional, remember to rotate your body so that different parts are exposed. If you already have a far-IR wood sauna, you could use the bulb fixture in there—but you don't have to turn on the far-IR sauna. You just use the four walls, ceiling, and floor. The same goes with the shower or other innovative enclosures that people can think of.

For maximum detoxification, as I've said, you need the air around you to be at least 100 degrees. Typically it's necessary to have an enclosure to ensure that level of heat, but depending on your environment or the time of year, your "sauna room" could be the size of a football stadium. If it's above 100 degrees, you could just sit in front of your four 250-watt, red-filtered, incandescent lamps anywhere you like.

What You Do After You Get Out of the Sauna Matters Too

After a sauna session, take a shower. You'll definitely want to wash off that toxic sweat and not leave it on your body to dry. To further maximize the benefits to your mitochondria, make it a cold shower.

Alternatively, you could take a cold plunge or swim in a cold pool. Ray Cronise, a former NASA scientist and diet researcher who has extensively studied the benefits of cold therapy, believes that the ideal temperature for cold thermogenesis, which has many mitochondrial benefits, is in the mid-60s and tolerable by most if you slowly work up to it.

You will need to have towels on hand to collect your sweat. Remember, you are sweating out real toxins and need to collect them unless your fixture is in a shower where you can rinse them down the drain.

How to Use a Sauna Safely

Moderate use of a sauna is safe for most people. However, if you have a heart condition, it is wise to consult with your physician first. Further precautions include:

- **Choose a low- or no-EMF near-infrared sauna.** If you are going to use an infrared sauna regularly, be sure you use one that emits low levels of electromagnetic fields (EMF); most models emit high levels of EMF. Look for one that emits low or no nonnative EMFs. You want to take care to research the levels of EMFs the sauna you use gives off, because in addition to causing cellular disturbances throughout the body, EMFs also activate your sympathetic nervous system, which will hamper your detox efforts.

    If you are purchasing a sauna, make sure the manufacturer supplies you with third-party spectral analysis that shows its levels of near infrared (in the 800 to 850 nanometer range) are just as high as the far infrared. Most saunas have far-infrared levels that are 20 times higher than near infrared. So be careful and do your homework before making an important health investment like a low-EMF full-spectrum infrared sauna. There are very few companies that sell an authentic near-IR sauna, and all the ones I know of have the incandescent heat lamp bulbs.

- **Stay safe.** Avoid using a sauna alone, as a sudden drop in blood pressure or dehydration may lead to a potentially lethal situation. Avoid the sauna if you are pregnant or if you are ill. Return to the sauna only after you are feeling better, don't have a fever, and are fully hydrated.

  Always listen to your body when deciding how much heat stress you can tolerate. If you've never used a sauna, you may need to start with just 4 minutes the first time, adding 30 seconds to each subsequent sauna until you reach 15 to 30 minutes. In some cases, the detoxification process may be severe. This schedule helps your body to slowly acclimate to sweating and eliminating toxins.

- **Avoid alcohol.** Alcohol in combination with sauna therapy increases your risk of arrhythmia, hypotension (extremely low blood pressure), dehydration, and sudden death. Studies from Finland, where sauna use is prevalent, found that those who experienced sudden death within 24 hours of using a sauna had a high probability of either consuming alcohol at the time or a history of chronic heavy drinking.[69, 70]

  Avoid the sauna if you've had too much to drink in the past 24 hours. While you may have heard sauna use will shorten a hangover, it actually increases your risk of dehydration at a time when you are already dehydrated from alcohol use.

- **Prevent dehydration and mineral loss.** Sauna use increases the amount of fluid you lose through sweating. It's important to replace that fluid by ensuring you are well hydrated with clean, pure water before using the sauna and paying close attention to rehydrating afterward.

For much more information, Dr. Lawrence Wilson's book *Sauna Therapy for Detoxification and Healing*, which I mentioned earlier in the chapter, is one of the better resources I've read on sauna use.

SUMMARY

- The environment and our food and water supplies are contaminated with huge numbers of persistent organic pollutants (POPs), which are fat-soluble and slow-to-degrade toxins.

- When ingested, your body will store POPs in fat cells in a defensive mechanism to protect the vital organs from toxic damage.

- When you fast, you burn fat stores; this releases fat-soluble toxins that have been stored in your fat cells, essentially reexposing you to high levels of toxins.

- In order to get liberated toxins out of your body, they need to be converted to a water-soluble form by the liver, and then excreted through urine, feces, or sweat.

- To facilitate the conversion to a water-soluble state, you need to have plenty of the nutrients that support your detoxification pathways on hand; you can do this by eating the high levels of low-net-carb vegetables, particularly cruciferous vegetables such as cauliflower and broccoli, which comprise the majority of the cyclical ketogenic diet.

- In addition to providing your body with detoxification-supporting foods, you can further boost your body's ability to detox harmful substances by drinking plenty of pure water, sweating, and taking fiber and other binders that will sweep the toxins out through the feces.

- To encourage passive sweating—which is more likely to contain toxins than sweat that's released when exercising—I recommend using a near-infrared sauna two to three times a week, and definitely on the day when you KetoFast.

CHAPTER 7

THE CYCLICAL KETOGENIC DIET

As powerful a health strategy as fasting is for weight loss and the improvement of so many markers of health, it's interesting to note that the long-term primary benefits are strongly influenced by the food you eat when you are not fasting.

This is because fasting is something that typically should only be done occasionally. Whether you're doing a partial fast on certain days or time-restrictive eating (TRE), it's not something you do continuously. Eating, on the other hand, is something that you do most every day. And the foods you eat will affect your health, for better or worse.

If you recall, TRE restricts the length of time each day when you can consume food to a small window that ranges from 6 to 8 hours, or up to 12 hours for practical purposes. Conventional TRE has no emphasis on the quality of food that is consumed during the hours that you can eat.

A 2018 study published in the journal *Nutrition and Healthy Aging* followed obese volunteers for three months.[1] The participants could eat as much as they wanted, and any food they wanted between the hours of 10 A.M. and 6 P.M. For the remaining

16 hours, they could have only water or calorie-free drinks. The outcomes of this eating strategy were then compared to a non-intervention control group from a previous fasting trial.

There were some surprisingly positive results for the 23 volunteers. The first is that they consumed about 350 fewer calories per day and lost just under 3 percent of their body weight. This study is the most convincing evidence I have seen against the common age-old "calories in, calories out" theory of weight loss.

However, many markers of health, such as visceral fat mass (a predictor of heart disease), diastolic blood pressure, LDL cholesterol, HDL cholesterol, triglycerides, fasting glucose, and fasting insulin, did not improve during this study. But can you imagine what the results would be if they had actually paid attention to the quality of the foods they ate during the study?

The study participants followed the standard American diet: A large portion of the food they consumed was processed, high in carbohydrates, sugars, damaged fats, and herbicides like glyphosate. Unless you move away from these types of foods and replace them with nutrient-dense unprocessed whole foods and balance your macronutrient ratios (a fancy way of saying get the right mix of carbs, protein, and fat in your diet), you might lose weight but otherwise not improve your health, as documented by the conventional tests mentioned above. If you lose weight but don't move the needle in the right direction for your glucose, insulin, and other disease-risk indicators, the benefit is little more than cosmetic.

In order to experience as many health benefits as possible from your fasting, you want to ensure that the diet you follow when you're not fasting lowers inflammation, normalizes insulin resistance, promotes mitochondrial health, maximizes cellular regeneration, and keeps aging in check. And this is precisely what following a cyclical ketogenic diet—or, in layman's terms, a fat-burning diet—can do.

But be careful, as even though intermittent fasting can have dramatic metabolic results such as reversing diabetes and obesity, it is similar to ketosis in that if you continue it indefinitely without breaking it up through partial fasting and days of higher carbs and protein during a compressed eating window, its benefits will often decrease and may even reverse.

WHY MAKING THE SWITCH TO BURNING FAT MATTERS

You may have heard the word *ketogenic* or had a friend tell you they were following a "keto" diet. It has become quite a buzzword, just as Paleo did before it. I wrote my previous book, *Fat for Fuel*, all about why and how to adopt a cyclical ketogenic diet, so if you want a deep dive, that book provides it. Here, I'll give you the CliffsNotes version.

A ketogenic diet is a high-fat, low-carb eating plan that has the goal of getting your body to be metabolically flexible—able to burn fat for fuel—as indicated by an ability to increase your production of ketones. If you recall, ketones are water-soluble fats made in your liver. When your body is able to produce them, you will experience profound changes that will push you in the direction of high-quality health. Ketones reduce oxidative stress by creating important antioxidants such as superoxide dismutase and catalase. They also create nicotinamide adenine dinucleotide phosphate (NADPH), a NAD coenzyme that recharges antioxidants like glutathione, ubiquinol, and vitamin C to a functional state.

WHAT IS METABOLIC FLEXIBILITY?

Metabolic flexibility is the ability to switch your body's primary energy source from carbs, in the form of glucose, to fat from fatty acid–derived ketones and stored fat. There is now a growing body of research indicating that ketones are the preferred fuel for both your brain and body during periods of fasting and extended exercise.[2, 3] When you are metabolically flexible, your body shifts from creating fat and storing it to actually using fat in the form of free fatty acids and ketones. For this reason, many experts have suggested that intermittent fasting regimens may have potential in the treatment of obesity and related metabolic conditions, including metabolic syndrome and type 2 diabetes.[4]

The switch to burning fat for fuel occurs when your liver glycogen stores are depleted and your body starts breaking down your fat stores to produce fatty acids and glycerol.[5] The metabolic shift typically occurs between 12 to 36 hours after you stop eating food, but could be longer if your liver has large glycogen stores from a high-carb diet. It is also influenced by your energy expenditure and amount of exercise, as higher expenditures will more rapidly deplete glycogen stores.

Once this shift occurs, the lipids in your fat cells (triacylglycerol and diacylglycerol) are metabolized to fatty acids, which are released into your blood. These fatty acids are then transported to your liver cells where they are converted by beta-oxidation to produce the ketones beta hydroxy butyrate (BOB) and acetoacetate, which perform their metabolic magic by increasing your mitochondrial function.[6] As I mentioned, one of the most important functions of ketones is that they reduce oxidative stress by increasing NADPH.[7, 8, 9]

The major biological functions of NADPH are threefold. The first is to act as a key component in recharging important antioxidants such as glutathione, vitamin E, and vitamin C. The second is to act as an electron source for synthesis of fatty acids, steroids,[10, 11] proteins, and DNA.[12] And the third is to act as the substrate for NADPH oxidase (NOX), which plays a key role in your immune function.

If you eat three or more meals per day without allowing your body time to recover, you simply won't flip your metabolic switch and you will likely never provide your body the ability to generate therapeutic ketone levels. Additionally, as your insulin resistance increases with excess weight and diabetes, the time it takes to get your body to the point where it can flip that metabolic switch will become progressively longer, as you see in the figure on page 93.

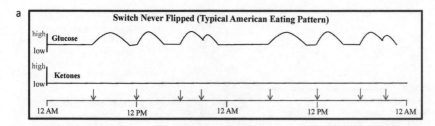

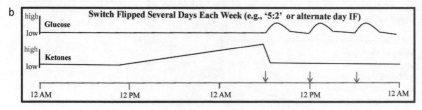

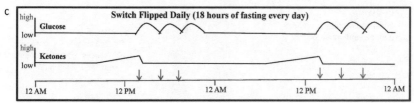

Profiles of circulating glucose and ketone levels over 48 hours in individuals with a typical American eating pattern or two different IF eating patterns. (a) In individuals who consume three meals plus snacks every day, the metabolic switch is never "flipped" and their ketone levels remain very low, and the area under the curve for glucose levels is high compared to individuals on an IF eating pattern. (b) In this example, the person fasted completely on the first day and then ate three separate meals on the subsequent day. On the fasting day ketones are progressively elevated and glucose levels remain low, whereas on the eating day ketones remain low and glucose levels are elevated during and for several hours following meal consumption. (c) In this example, the person consumes all of their food within a 6-hour time window every day. Thus, the metabolic switch is flipped on following 12 hours of fasting and remains on for approximately 6 hours each day, until food is consumed after approximately 18 hours of fasting.

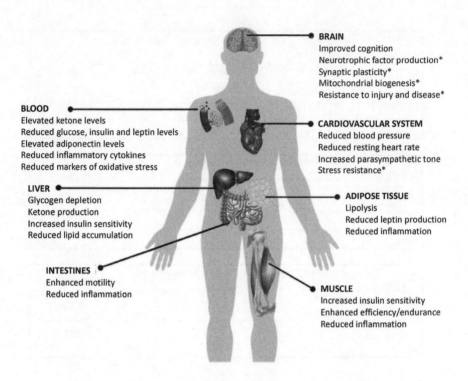

BRAIN
Improved cognition
Neurotrophic factor production*
Synaptic plasticity*
Mitochondrial biogenesis*
Resistance to injury and disease*

BLOOD
Elevated ketone levels
Reduced glucose, insulin and leptin levels
Elevated adiponectin levels
Reduced inflammatory cytokines
Reduced markers of oxidative stress

CARDIOVASCULAR SYSTEM
Reduced blood pressure
Reduced resting heart rate
Increased parasympathetic tone
Stress resistance*

LIVER
Glycogen depletion
Ketone production
Increased insulin sensitivity
Reduced lipid accumulation

ADIPOSE TISSUE
Lipolysis
Reduced leptin production
Reduced inflammation

INTESTINES
Enhanced motility
Reduced inflammation

MUSCLE
Increased insulin sensitivity
Enhanced efficiency/endurance
Reduced inflammation

Examples of functional effects and major cellular and molecular responses of various organ systems to IF. In humans and rodents, IF results in decreased levels of circulating insulin and leptin, elevated ketone levels, and reduced levels of pro-inflammatory cytokines and markers of oxidative stress. Liver cells respond to fasting by generating ketones and by increasing insulin sensitivity and decreasing lipid accumulation. Markers of inflammation in the intestines are reduced by IF. The insulin sensitivity of muscle cells is enhanced and inflammation reduced in muscle cells in response to the metabolic switch triggered by fasting and exercise. Emerging findings further suggest that exercise training in the fasted state may enhance muscle growth and endurance. Robust beneficial effects of IF on the cardiovascular system have been documented, including reduced blood pressure, reduced resting heart rate, increased heart rate variability (improved cardiovascular stress adaptation), and resistance of cardiac muscle to damage in animal models of myocardial infarction. Studies of laboratory animals and human subjects have shown that IF can improve cognition (learning and memory): the underlying mechanisms may involve neurotrophic factors, stimulation of mitochondrial biogenesis and autophagy, and the formation of new synapses. IF also increases the resistance of neurons to stress and suppresses neuroinflammation.

*Demonstrated in animal models, but not yet evaluated in humans.

Compared to an eating pattern in which food is consumed from the time you wake up to the time you go to bed (12 or more hours daily), intermittent fasting eating patterns may result in a wide range of beneficial effects on health, including improved glucose metabolism,[13, 14, 15, 16, 17] reduced inflammation,[18, 19] reduced blood pressure,[20] improved cardiovascular health,[21, 22] and increased resistance of cells to stress and disease (see figure on page 94).[23, 24, 25]

In a study of 34 healthy men randomly assigned to either a normal control diet or daily TRE (16 hours of daily fasting) and followed for two months during which they maintained a standard resistance-training program, the men in the TRE group showed a reduction in fat mass with retention of lean mass and maximal strength.[26]

There are many studies done with TRE, and some participants experience difficulties adhering to the protocol.[27, 28, 29, 30, 31] However, surprisingly few studies documented where participants actually made the switch and were able to create ketones, which makes it imperative to confirm that you are actually in nutritional ketosis. You can easily confirm this with ketone test strips or objective labs to prevent these difficulties.

When you follow a cyclical ketogenic diet, you enter nutritional ketosis—the biological state of being able to burn fat, defined as having blood ketones in the range of 0.5 to 3.0 millimoles per liter (mmol/L). You can detect the presence of ketones in your body with a device that measures the ketones in your blood, such as Keto-Mojo, or your breath, using Ketonix, or in your urine, with a wide variety of inexpensive ketone test strips.

GLUCOSE VS. KETONES

Your cells use glucose, which is a sugar that is produced either by your liver, in a process called gluconeogenesis, the formation of glucose by the liver from precursors other than carbs, especially from amino acids (protein) and glycerol from fats, or during the metabolic process after eating foods that contain carbohydrates. If you indulge regularly in some form of the high-carb, ultra-processed standard American diet that includes bagels, sandwiches, pasta, fast food, and chips, you are almost assuredly burning glucose as your primary source of fuel and are not metabolically flexible.

Glucose is not an ideal fuel for your body to run on exclusively for a few reasons, the primary one being that when your cells use glucose as their primary fuel, they produce excess reactive oxygen species (ROS), which, as we learned in Chapter 1, are a significant source of oxidative stress that contributes to most diseases, including premature aging. Healthy fats, on the other hand, create far fewer ROS than glucose when burned. In other words, fat is a far cleaner-burning fuel than glucose.

Another major problem with excessive glucose consumption is that it increases insulin resistance. Insulin resistance is worsened when your blood sugar spikes several times a day—such as when you have excessive carbs at every meal, like a bagel for breakfast, sandwich for lunch, and pasta for dinner, with one or more sugary treats thrown in. Whether it's a specialty coffee drink, a cookie, or full-on dessert (or all three), your body produces more and more insulin in response, and over time, your insulin receptors become progressively more resistant.

Additionally, your body has a strict limit on the amount of glucose it can store. First it converts glucose to glycogen and then stashes away as much of it as it can in your liver or in your muscles. However, the capacity to store glycogen is limited in most people to one or two pounds. This is in stark contrast to the virtually unlimited capacity to store fat, which could be hundreds of pounds in some individuals.

If you are not fat-adapted and your glycogen stores run low, you will experience pressing hunger pangs, which is your body's attempt to get you to feed it more glucose. Since your body has a practically unlimited ability to store fat, if you are metabolically flexible and have captured the ability to burn fat for fuel, you can go long periods without eating and experience little to no hunger, making your daily life and the times when you opt to fast from food far easier.

BENEFITS OF NUTRITIONAL KETOSIS

When you help your body restore its ability to create and then use ketones as another source of fuel, you experience a wide array of benefits—some of which you'll be able to feel and some of which are happening beneath the level of your awareness. Either way, the ketones your liver makes are working hard to produce many positive effects including:

- **Improved insulin sensitivity.** When you are in nutritional ketosis, your blood glucose levels naturally fall because you are not continually eating carbohydrates, which tend to raise your glucose level. As a result, your body needs to produce less insulin, which gives your insulin receptors a chance to regain their sensitivity to insulin. Studies have shown that diabetics who stick to a ketogenic diet are able to significantly reduce their dependency on diabetic medications. Many have even successfully reversed their diabetes this way.[32] Having less insulin resistance will also lower your risk for Alzheimer's, as dementia and insulin resistance are closely linked.[33]

- **Reduced inflammation.** When you burn ketones for fuel, far fewer ROS are created. Additionally, ketones are very powerful histone deacetylase inhibitors (HDAC) that will reduce inflammatory cytokines and cause your body to produce many natural anti-inflammatories. So, by optimizing the amount of carbs in your diet and nudging your body into nutritional ketosis, you significantly decrease your risk of chronic inflammation—a precursor to nearly every chronic disease.

- **Reduced risk of cancer.** Unlike your regular cells, cancer cells lack the metabolic flexibility to use ketones for their energy needs. That means that once your body enters nutritional ketosis, cancer cells no longer have a source of fuel. This will help not only prevent many cancers, but also will be an important resource in an effective supplemental strategy to treat cancer.

- **Increased longevity.** Ketosis helps clear out malfunctioning immune cells[34] and plays an important role in autophagy (the recycling of damaged cellular components that occurs within your cells) and mitophagy (the digestion and removal of the entire mitochondria). It does this by inhibiting the mTOR pathway. As a result, ketosis improves your overall mitochondria function, which will go far in preventing and treating nearly every chronic degenerative disease.

  A ketogenic diet is very low in sugar, which is a potent accelerator of aging and premature death, in part because it activates two genes—Ras and PKA— that are known to accelerate aging.[35]

- **Weight loss.** Once you're fat-adapted and metabolically flexible, whenever your glycogen stores run low, your body will tap into its fat stores for energy, which helps with fat loss.

  The near disappearance of hunger and food cravings when you are fat-adapted also helps you maintain that weight loss once you're at an ideal weight. In one study,[36] obese test subjects were given either a low-carb ketogenic diet or a low-fat diet. After 24 weeks, researchers noted that the low-carb group lost more weight (9.4 kilograms; 20.7 pounds) compared to the low-fat group (4.8 kilograms; 10.5 pounds).

- **Mental clarity.** One of the best benefits of ketones is that they are a preferred fuel for your brain. So, once you start using them for brain function, you pave the way for improved mental clarity. In fact, one of the first things many people notice once they start burning fat for fuel is that any "brain fog" lifts, and they regain the mental clarity they had when they were much younger and healthier.

HOW TO EAT FOR KETOSIS

In general, the way to achieve nutritional ketosis is to reduce the number of net carbs you eat—a measurement you can determine by subtracting the number of grams of fiber in a food from the total number of carbohydrates—and replace those calories with high-quality fats and low-starch vegetables. As a general rule, you'll want to keep your net carbs to a maximum of 20 to 50 grams or fewer a day.

It's also important that you restrict your protein intake to an adequate amount. You basically want to consume only as much protein as your body needs to maintain your muscle mass, and no more.

Why?

Because any excess protein is a strong stimulus for the mTOR pathway, which is a powerful catabolic signal that will tend to raise your glucose levels. The formula for determining your target protein intake for a day is to calculate your lean body mass in kilograms, and then eat one gram of protein for every kilogram of lean body mass. If you are imperially oriented to the U.S. measuring system, a close approximation is to target one-half gram of protein for every pound of lean body mass.

However, as you get older, your body requires additional protein to maintain your body mass. So your needs would increase by about 25 percent. Additionally, athletes and pregnant women need to increase their protein intake by anywhere from 25 to 50 percent.

If you are older than 65 and you exercise regularly, you will likely need to increase your protein intake by 50 percent on days you exercise. This is even more important if you are doing extensive cardio, which seems to further increase protein requirements. This will help prevent age-related loss of muscle tissue, known as sarcopenia.

In order to reap the most benefits of the cyclical ketogenic diet, you want to eliminate packaged, processed foods. To make sure you're meeting your nutritional requirements and maintaining the ideal nutrient ratios, use a free online nutrient tracker such as Cronometer (www.cronometer.com/mercola), which is already set up for nutritional ketosis.

A WORD ABOUT THE FATS YOU SHOULD BE EATING—AND THE ONES YOU SHOULDN'T

This is probably a far higher-fat diet than you are used to, which makes it even more important to select the right fats, as not all fats are created equal. Ideally, you'll forgo all industrially processed vegetable oils used in processed foods and fried restaurant meals as much as possible because they will wreak havoc on your mitochondrial health. It will be important to prioritize high-quality healthy fats, including:

- Olives and olive oil (preferably third-party-certified olive oil to ensure it hasn't been adulterated with lower-quality vegetable oils)

- Coconuts and coconut oil (excellent for cooking as it can withstand higher temperatures without oxidizing; be sure to buy a product labeled "hexane-free" and "chemical-free" so that your healthy coconut oil doesn't deliver toxins along with its good fats)

- Animal-based omega-3 fat from fatty fish low in mercury, such as wild-caught Alaskan salmon, sardines, anchovies, herring and/or krill oil

- Butter, preferably made from raw, grass-fed, organic milk

- Raw nuts that aren't too high in protein, such as macadamias and pecans

- Avocados

- Seeds such as black sesame, black cumin, pumpkin, and hemp

- Grass-fed meats

- Ghee (clarified butter), lard, and tallow (excellent for cooking)
- Raw cacao butter
- Organic, pastured egg yolks
- Medium-chain triglyceride (MCT) oil

DRAWBACKS OF LONG-TERM KETOSIS

While eating a ketogenic diet and being metabolically flexible are beneficial for your overall health, and specifically your mitochondrial health, long-term, or even worse, continuous ketosis is generally not a wise strategy. There are a few reasons why this is so.

Insulin Levels Fall Too Low

Paradoxically, long-term uninterrupted use of a ketogenic diet can trigger a rise in your blood sugar by driving your insulin levels too low. It turns out one of the primary functions of insulin is to suppress gluconeogenesis—the process your liver uses to produce glucose. The reason this is not widely appreciated is that very few people actually have insulin levels low enough to stop their liver's production of glucose. About the only times this happens is during prolonged fasting and continuous noncyclical nutritional ketosis with low-net-carb intakes.

When your insulin levels remain consistently low, your liver gets the signal to start ramping up glucose production, because your body assumes you must be going into starvation mode and it is seeking to provide enough glucose to fuel your brain. While your brain can run primarily on ketones and fats, it requires a minimum of around 15 percent glucose to function properly. If you aren't providing glucose directly through your diet, your body cues your liver to produce it.

If you continue fasting too long, your metabolism will shift to breaking down muscle in order to hold on to fat stores, meaning you'll become vulnerable to losing muscle mass and gaining fat if you remain in uninterrupted low-carb consumption for too long. Fortunately there are very simple strategies you can implement to prevent this from ever happening.

What is really counterintuitive is that when you are in a low-insulin, elevated-blood-glucose state and you eat a small amount of carbs, your blood sugar will actually drop! This is because the carbohydrates you ate were enough to raise insulin levels, which then stopped the gluconeogenesis process.

When seeking to understand why low insulin has this result, it can be helpful to consider that your body is programmed to survive in all kinds of dire conditions. If it feels your fat stores are running too low, or that there aren't enough carbohydrate calories to sustain you, it will shift into breaking down muscle tissue in order to produce glucose so that you don't have to run through all your fat stores. After all, your body believes, you may need those fat stores someday, and perhaps sooner than you think. So why not sacrifice a little muscle in the name of staying alive?

I have spoken with many clinicians who employ cyclical ketosis as a therapeutic strategy, and they confirm that many of their patients who spend an extended time in ketosis begin to lose muscle and gain fat. If you experience this phenomenon, you are likely to notice a lack of energy as well as weight that is difficult to lose.

Lack of Variety

Variety is a deeply important biological principle. Using one form of exercise or diet exclusively for long periods of time is likely to cause unintended adverse health consequences, no matter how useful the diet or exercise is. Your body evolved to be able to adapt, but if you never change your inputs, you are no longer forced to adapt. Ancient cultures strengthened their survival mechanisms naturally through seasonal dietary changes and environmental factors that impacted their food supply.[37] Today, with our year-round access to all manner of foods, we are no longer forced to cycle naturally and have this type of dietary variation.

By continually requiring your metabolism to adapt to new dietary patterns, you increase hormone sensitivity, raise growth hormone levels, support brain function,[38] and strengthen your microbiome. For these reasons, it is wise to integrate variety and cycling into your food plan after you have regained your ability to burn fat as your primary fuel.

I have also found that regular variation in diet helps encourage long-term compliance to a healthy lifestyle because periodically changing up what you eat helps ward off feelings of frustration, deprivation, and boredom with the same foods.

Lacks the Benefits of Feasting

Nutritional ketosis shares many of the same benefits of fasting—reduced blood sugar levels, improved insulin sensitivity, and improved mitochondrial health chief among them. But many of the upsides of fasting don't present themselves while you're going without food, but rather when you reintroduce food once your fast is over.

This is called the refeeding phase, which reminds your body it's not starving, stops the breakdown of muscle, reignites fat burning, and uses the stress from the fast to make you far healthier than you could have been without it. This is very similar to exercise in which you actually damage your tissues but during the recovery phase become much stronger and fitter than you were without it.

From a metabolic perspective, clearance of damaged cells and damaged cellular components occurs during fasting, while the rebuilding of cells and tissues occurs during the refeeding phase. In other words, cells and tissues are rebuilt and restored to a healthier state during refeeding. And when you stay in ketosis and never come back out, you aren't able to benefit from the refeeding phase.

Research has shown that fasting actually triggers the regeneration of the pancreas in both type 2 and, surprisingly, type 1 diabetics.[39] But again, these regenerative effects are largely triggered during the refeeding phase.

CYCLICAL KETOSIS TO THE RESCUE

The way I recommend addressing all these potential down-sides of extended ketosis is to alternate between "feast" and "famine" days in what I call cyclical ketosis. When you use this approach, you approximate the eating pattern of your ancient ancestors who did not have access to the same foods every day, and naturally had to adapt to some days when they ate more and many days when they ate far less or nothing at all.

Once you are able to burn fat for fuel (as shown by measuring your ketone production over 0.5 mmol/L), you can begin implementing cyclical ketosis. Once you have been in ketosis for at least a month, begin adding in one or two "feast days" per week, while eating your regular ketogenic diet on the other days. On these days, allow yourself to eat more net carbs and more protein. You should also reduce your fat intake on these days to make up for the extra carb and protein calories you're consuming. Ideally it would be best to schedule feast days for when you are engaging in vigorous exercise, so that your body can use the extra calories from carbs and protein to rebuild stronger muscles.

After a few days of feasting, you then cycle back into nutritional ketosis (the fasting stage). By periodically having days of higher carb intakes—consuming 100 or 150 grams of carbs as opposed to 20 to 50 grams per day, for example—your ketone levels will increase dramatically, your blood sugar will drop, your muscle mass will be spared, and your innate desire for dietary variety will be satisfied. If done prudently, this will not impair your body's ability to burn fat.

Once you have established yourself in a regular cyclical ketosis eating pattern, you can even increase and accelerate the health benefits by adding in periodic partial fasts (I guide you through exactly how to do that in Chapter 8). To get started, though, make it your goal to implement cyclical ketosis as outlined below. The rest can come when you and your physiology are ready.

I know that just the sound of the phrase "feast day" may conjure up images of hitting an all-you-can-eat buffet or gorging on everything in sight. Unfortunately, I'm afraid food quality still matters. While you can certainly increase your carb and protein intake on these days, you still want to avoid processed and junk foods. You want highly nutritious foods, just in different ratios of macronutrients than on your typical keto-friendly days.

These are the guidelines you'll want to follow on your feast days:

Increase Your Carbs

On feast days, you can triple your intake of healthy forms of carbs to within the range of 100 to 150 grams or so. You still want to eat plenty of vegetables on your feast days, but you can also add in other carb-rich foods that aren't typically part of a ketogenic diet, such as fruits, sweet potatoes, purple potatoes (my current favorite), rice, and quinoa. There are certain types of foods that are healthier for you than others, such as sweet potatoes (ideally cooled after initially cooking and reheated), underripe bananas, papayas, and mangoes, because they are high in digestive-resistant starches that can't be utilized by the human body but that feed the good bacteria in your gut.

Digestive-resistant starches are low-viscous fibers that resist digestion in the small intestine, add significant bulk to your stools, and help you stay regular. They also slowly ferment in your large intestine.[40] (Don't worry, the fermentation process is very slow, so they won't make you gassy.) Interestingly, by-products of this fermentation process in your gut are short-chain fatty acids that actually get converted to ketones by your gut bacteria and liver. This helps reduce inflammation, improve immune function,[41] normalize blood pressure,[42, 43, 44] and lower your risk of heart disease and heart attack.[45]

Best of all, since most of these carbs are indigestible, resistant starches do not result in blood sugar or insulin spikes. In fact, research suggests that resistant starches help improve insulin regulation, reducing your risk of insulin resistance.[46, 47, 48] Science also suggests resistant starch may play a role in the prevention of colon cancer[49] and inflammatory bowel disease.[50]

My favorite rice is organic white basmati, simply because I think it tastes the best. You might be surprised that I'm recommending a white rice, but it actually has far fewer problematic lectins (natural plant compounds found in the seeds, skins, and hulls of many fruits and vegetables that cause inflammation in the gut when consumed) than brown rice, and the minimal additional fiber in brown rice is easily replaced with other foods.

Basmati rice has a fair amount of resistant starch in it no matter how you cook it, but when you cook it, cool it, and then reheat it, that content goes up even more. Even better, a study has found that when you cook rice with a teaspoon of coconut oil added to the water and then cool the rice for 12 hours, the resistant starch is increased tenfold and calories reduced by as much as 60 percent.[51] (Remember to be sure that your coconut oil is hexane- and chemical-free.)

Interestingly, even bread can be made healthier through heating and cooling. According to a 2008 study published in the *European Journal of Clinical Nutrition*,[52] eating bread that had been frozen, defrosted, and/or toasted resulted in significantly lower blood glucose measurements than eating either homemade or commercial bread fresh out of the oven. I still recommend avoiding wheat because it is often contaminated by glyphosate, and even if it's organic and whole wheat, it still contains lectins— natural plant compounds that can cause gut inflammation when consumed. But I understand that some may love a perfect piece of toast. If you do decide to include bread on your feast days, make sure it is organic, white, and preferably sourdough bread (since the fermentation process reduces most of the gluten content) that has been frozen or refrigerated and then toasted.

Eat More Protein

You also need to increase your protein intake on feast days, but it would be wise to synchronize this with the days you are strength training so you can take advantage of the anabolic boost that is provided by activating the mTOR pathway with additional protein. It would also be wise to limit the amount to approximately double your normal protein intake, but you can play around with increasing it up to three times.

It is important to remember that in most cases, you should avoid exceeding 25 grams of protein (35 grams if you are a large, muscular male) in one meal, as that will likely exceed your body's ability to effectively use the amino acids and will simply put an extra burden on your kidneys. So be careful to space your protein intake throughout your day.

Reduce Your Fat Intake

On feast days, you'll want to reduce your fat consumption so that you don't end up consuming too many calories—after all, you will be eating considerably more calories from carbs on these days, and perhaps more protein too. You have to even out the equation somewhere, and fat is where you'll do it.

Continue to Avoid Eating for at Least Three Hours before Bedtime

As I explained in Chapter 1, I believe that everyone—no matter their state of health or eating plan—benefits immensely from refraining from eating within three hours of bedtime so that your body gets ample time to digest your meal before going into rest mode. The same is true even on feast days.

In Chapter 8, I'll go into greater detail on how to build on the benefits of a cyclical ketogenic diet by incorporating regular time-restricted eating and partial fasting in what I now believe to be the very best eating strategy for just about everyone.

Also, remember, for much more information on how and why to get into ketosis, refer to my book *Fat for Fuel*, and for nearly 100 delicious and keto-compliant recipes, pick up the *Fat for Fuel Ketogenic Cookbook* that I wrote in tandem with world-class healthy chef Pete Evans.

SUMMARY

- A ketogenic diet is a high-fat, low-carb eating plan that has the goal of triggering your body to regain the ability to burn fat for fuel as indicated by an increased level of ketones.

- Ketones are water-soluble fats made in your liver that supply you with energy after your reserves of glycogen —the stored form of glucose—are depleted.

- Metabolic flexibility is the ability to easily switch between using glucose and fat for fuel; most people lost their metabolic flexibility decades ago because of a focus on high-carb diets and never going more than a few hours without food while awake.

- A ketogenic diet is a low-carb, high-fat, adequate-protein diet that encourages your body to enter a state of ketosis.

- Being in constant ketosis for long periods of time can be highly counterproductive long term, and will typically lead to a loss of many of its initial benefits; to remedy this, I recommend adding in one or two days when you eat more carbs and protein in what I call cyclical ketosis once metabolic flexibility has been achieved.

- The high-carb, higher-protein days—or what I call feast days—of a cyclical ketogenic diet spur a cascade of health benefits that you don't enjoy if you consistently follow a ketogenic diet that *doesn't* include feast days, as the feast days are when your body rebuilds itself.

- On your feast days, increase your carb intake from 20 to 50 grams of healthy carbs to 120 to 150 grams, double your daily protein allotment, and reduce your fat intake (so that you don't end up overconsuming calories).

CHAPTER 8

HOW TO KETOFAST

Now that you know all the reasons to restore your metabolic flexibility and begin engaging in regular partial fasting, all you need are the specifics on exactly *how* to do so.

Before we dive in, it's important to remember to pay attention to your body as you implement each step, and only progress to the next phase when you feel you have adjusted. If you are generally healthy when you begin this process, you can likely move through the steps fairly rapidly. If you are facing health challenges, including excess weight or insulin resistance—which up to 80 percent of Americans have—you will want to give yourself more time to progress through the steps according to your tolerance.

If you are taking any medications, it will also be wise to have your health-care practitioner monitor your prescriptions during this process. KetoFasting will help you eliminate medications you might be taking for high blood pressure or high cholesterol, but you will need to be carefully supervised in this process to prevent any complications.

At the end of this chapter, you'll find a "How to KetoFast" quick-reference chart that will make it easy for you to apply what you've learned.

BEFORE YOU START:
MINIMIZE YOUR TOXIC EXPOSURE

While KetoFasting is a powerful tool to help you eliminate the toxins that you are exposed to, it really is the last step of a comprehensive approach to reducing your toxic exposure. While you certainly can do KetoFasting without implementing the steps I describe here and receive benefit, if you do them, you will optimize your time and effort.

The first step you can take to aid your body's detoxification process and limit any side effects is to radically limit your toxin load by avoiding as many toxins as you can. Limit your use of chemicals in your household cleaners and your personal care products, including cosmetics, as these items are typically loaded with chemicals.

It's also important to drink pure, filtered water and avoid plastic water bottles, which can be loaded with hormone disruptors like BPA and phthalates. You'll also want to avoid drinking hot beverages from Styrofoam cups.

Other commonly overlooked sources of toxic exposure include mercury (silver) fillings, airplane travel, scented candles, and vehicle emissions. For more information, the Environmental Working Group's website (www.EWG.org) is a great repository of guidance on choosing nontoxic products.

Infections in your gut, such as small intestinal bowel overgrowth (SIBO), can also be an issue by contributing to the release of infectious toxins such as lipopolysaccharides (LPS). This is often best addressed by specific dietary adjustments, which remove prebiotic beneficial fibers that could be feeding these organisms, otherwise known as the low-FODMAP diet. This restricted diet is only done until the SIBO resolves, at which point you can progress to wider food options offered by *Fat for Fuel* and *KetoFast*.

The next step is to remediate your personal nutritional biochemistry pathways and nutrient deficiencies. The best place to start is to find a knowledgeable clinician who has used urinary organic acid testing. This test measures the organic acids excreted in your urine and can highlight how well your avenues of detoxification are working, such as your liver and the methylation process. It can also predict the presence of SIBO, illuminate how well your body is burning fat, and point out nutritional deficiencies such as vitamin B_{12}. The test will also help uncover genetic defects that may be affecting you and your mitochondrial functions.

My favorite lab for this is Great Plains; it provides an in-home test that only requires you to submit a urine specimen, although you do need a physician to authorize your request for a testing kit to be sent to you. The clinic I personally use to review the results of the test is run by Bob Miller, N.D., at https://www.tolhealth.com/. Consultations can be done over the phone.

You also want to make sure that you are having daily bowel movements before engaging in KetoFasting, because if you are constipated you won't be able to effectively release the toxins through your stool and they will likely be resorbed. Shifting to a cyclical ketogenic diet will get your digestion moving again as you implement the early stages of the program.

BEGIN EATING ONLY ORGANIC FOODS

The most impactful way to radically reduce your toxic exposures is by choosing foods that aren't grown with poisonous pesticides—in other words, eating organic produce whenever possible—and sticking to purely organic meat and dairy, as they tend to concentrate toxins far more than vegetables.

You may feel that eating organic is too expensive, but when you look at the long-term cost of choosing foods with residues of harmful pesticides, I think you'll agree that the higher price tag is more than worth it.

Are organic foods healthier and therefore worth the extra expense? If "healthier" means the absence of herbicide and pesticide contamination and higher nutrient content, then the answer is yes. A meta-analysis[1] published by researchers at Stanford University in 2012 looked at 240 studies comparing organically and conventionally grown food, and confirmed that organics were 23 to 37 percent less likely to contain detectable pesticide residues. Organically raised chicken was also up to 45 percent less likely to contain antibiotic-resistant bacteria.

Following in Stanford University's footsteps, a group of scientists at Newcastle University in the U.K. evaluated an even greater number of studies—343 in all, published over several decades. Just like the Stanford study, their follow-up analysis,[2] published in 2014, found that while conventional and organic vegetables oftentimes offer similar levels of many nutrients, organic fruits and vegetables were found to contain anywhere from 18 to 69 percent more antioxidants than conventionally grown varieties.

Additionally, the frequency of occurrence of pesticide residues was four times higher in conventional foods. Conventional produce also had on average 48 percent higher levels of cadmium, a toxic metal and a known carcinogen.[3]

There are a number of other studies that support the claim that organically grown produce contains higher levels of nutrients in general. For example, a study[4] partially funded by the U.S. Department of Agriculture (USDA) found that organic strawberries were more nutrient-rich than conventional strawberries. Interestingly, a recent study showed that strawberries are high in a polyphenol called fisetin, which is useful in removing senescent cells from your body.[5] Senescent cells are cells that have stopped reproducing either due to age or oxidative damage and tend to clog up your metabolic machinery. There is much exciting new longevity research that shows that removing senescent cells extends lifespan.

When it comes to eating organic food, you also want to choose organic dairy and meat. Two 2016 studies, one on the compositional differences of organic and conventional meat,[6] and one on dairy,[7] found clear differences between the two—primarily, that organic milk and meat had significantly more omega-3 fatty acids and fewer omega-6 fatty acids than their conventional counterparts. In one of the largest efforts of its kind, researchers analyzed 196 and 67 studies on dairy and meat respectively.

Research has also found that true organic free-range (pastured) eggs typically contain about two-thirds more vitamin A, double the amount of omega-3, three times more vitamin E, and as much as seven times more beta carotene than conventional eggs.[8]

Choosing organic is also extremely important to the health of our environment. Many pesticides biodegrade very slowly, if at all, and remain in the environment for years. To make matters worse, some chemicals used to treat crops, such as pendimethalin, can remain airborne for weeks on end, practically ensuring pesticide drift that contaminates the broader environment as well as neighboring farms. Depending on wind conditions during spraying, the chemicals can travel long distances, contaminating organic fields where such pesticides are not legal to use. It's a lot like secondhand smoke: If a nonsmoker is sitting next to someone who lights up, the nonsmoker ends up inhaling toxins even though he or she has made the choice to live a healthier lifestyle.

If you want to know which conventionally grown fruits and vegetables carry the greatest toxic load in terms of pesticides, the Environmental Working Group (EWG)[9] provides a list of the worst offenders, called the "Dirty Dozen." These are among the most important foods to buy organic. They update the list every year, and you can visit their site to find the latest list. The foods on the 2018 list are:

1. Strawberries
2. Spinach
3. Nectarines
4. Apples
5. Grapes
6. Peaches
7. Cherries
8. Pears
9. Tomatoes
10. Celery
11. Potatoes
12. Sweet bell peppers

EWG also lists plant-based foods considered to be the safest bets to purchase conventionally grown, as they generally have the lowest amount of pesticide spray residue. These are known as the "Clean 15":

1. Avocados
2. Sweet corn
3. Pineapple
4. Cabbage
5. Onions
6. Sweet peas, frozen
7. Papaya
8. Asparagus
9. Mango
10. Eggplant
11. Honeydew melon
12. Kiwi
13. Cantaloupe
14. Cauliflower
15. Broccoli

If organic foods are simply unattainable where you live, one way to minimize potential ill effects from eating heavily sprayed produce is to peel fruits and vegetables, such as sweet potatoes and apples, whenever possible. But recognize that this is a poor second choice as apple peels are loaded with important and beneficial phytochemicals and likely far more important for your health than the actual fruit. So if you can, seek out organic, and eat the peel to get maximum benefits.

Unless you can find an organic restaurant, you'll want to limit eating out to avoid their conventional produce, dairy, and meat. In general, the only way to ensure the quality and nutrition of your food is to buy and prepare it yourself at home.

As important as it is to eat organic foods whenever possible, it's even more important to eat them on your partial fast days when you will be in fat-burning mode, only eating 300 to 600 calories and, therefore, more exposed to toxins that have been released from your fat cells.

KETOFASTING STEP BY STEP

Step One: Stop Eating Three Hours Before Bedtime

I covered this extensively in Chapter 1, but I can't emphasize it enough: Remember to stop eating and drinking anything other than water within the three hours before bedtime. This will give your body more of a chance to digest the food you eat before you go to sleep, reduce oxidative damage, optimize your mitochondrial function, and devote more energy to detoxification and repair while you are sleeping.

Step Two: Reduce Your Eating Window with Time-Restricted Eating

Once you have adjusted and are comfortable to going without food for the three hours before bedtime, work to reduce your window of eating until you are fasting 16 to 18 hours each day and eating only during a time span of 6 to 8 hours a day—for example, eating only between 11 A.M. and 7 P.M. (for an 8-hour window) or noon and 6 P.M. (for a 6-hour window).

Even without changing the foods that you eat during your eating window, prolonging the number of hours when you aren't eating will help your body become more metabolically flexible and give it more time for detoxification and repair than it normally gets when you eat at all hours of the day.

It may take anywhere between a week and a month or two to get to the point where you can comfortably go up to 18 hours between your last meal of the day and the first meal of the next day. Just keep in mind that eight of those hours you will be sleeping, and three of those hours will be the hours before bed. By 7 A.M., you already have 12 hours behind you and you just need to delay your first meal till 11 A.M. for 16 hours or 1 P.M. for 18 hours.

Step Three: Make the Switch to a Cyclical Ketogenic Diet

In order for KetoFast to work, your body needs regain the ability to burn fat as a primary fuel. For specific guidance on exactly how to do this, see Chapter 7 in this book, as well as my previous book, *Fat for Fuel*. But essentially, cut way back on your carbs and replace them with healthy fats.

Make sure that you eat plenty of nutrient-dense foods on your ketogenic diet. A simple principle you can use is to avoid packaged, processed foods and replace them with real organic foods. This might mean you're buying foods that cost more, and it may also take more of your time to prepare than quick and convenient processed foods, but the upside is that it will keep you healthy, and radically reduce your visits to the doctor and hospital.

To know for sure that you've regained your ability to burn fat for fuel, you'll want to monitor your ketone levels. To do that, you'll need some kind of a device, as outlined below.

Ketone Monitoring Devices and Accessories

There are three ways to measure your body's ketone output:

- **Blood test.** The simple and easy way to see if you are in nutritional ketosis is to measure your blood levels of beta-hydroxybutyrate (BHB; a form of ketone). You'll know you are in ketosis when they are between 0.5 and 3.0 mmol/L.

  My favorite ketone device and the one I use is Keto-Mojo. The major benefit is that the Mojo's measuring strips are only $1 each, which is a fraction of the prices of the other meters. Other options I've seen cost around $4 to $6 *per strip*.

- **Breathalyzer.** These devices measure the acetone in your breath. Acetone is the substance that BHB breaks down into, and is an indicator of the amount of BHB present in the blood. You simply blow into the meter for 20 to 30 seconds and it will flash one of three different colors a specific number of times to indicate your level of ketosis. Ketonix.com sells its version for $150—but the advantage is that you don't need to pay for testing strips, and you don't have to draw any blood.

- **Urine test.** For many decades, urine test strips that measure the presence of acetoacetate (another type of ketone) have been the most common way to measure ketosis. The reactive pad at the end of the strips remains beige if there are no ketones present and turns pink with light ketones and purple for strong ketones.

But since they only detect acetoacetate and not BHB, which is the fuel preferred by most cells, urine tests provide limited insight into whether your body is actually burning fat for fuel. On the other hand, they're inexpensive, fairly convenient to use, and don't require pricking your finger. You can use the strips simply to see if your body is producing ketones (any level of pink color means that it is).

When to Monitor Ketones

Although it's helpful to know when your body is producing ketones, it's not necessary to test them regularly or on a continuous basis. It's all too easy to become obsessed with your levels, and I would rather you focus on eating high-quality foods and enhancing your detoxification abilities.

However, when you change your eating or partial fasting schedule or your diet, it is always great to see if your liver is still making ketones or if you have somehow self-sabotaged. To help you know when it's worth the time and expense of checking in on your ketone levels, here are some guidelines:

- **When you first begin a ketogenic diet.** You really only need to monitor your ketones closely at the beginning of your KetoFast journey. Doing so can provide you with important feedback in two areas: First, it will help you determine when you have successfully made the transition to burning fat; second, it will help you fine-tune your personal limit on how many and what kind of carbs you can eat and still remain in that fat-burning state. It can take some fine-tuning of your diet to get your ketone levels into the range of 0.5 to 3.0 mmol/L, and monitoring your ketone levels can give you some very important quantifiable data on how well your plan is working.

- **To determine your carb threshold level.** To get an accurate picture of how many carbs you can eat and still produce ample ketones, you'll want to stick to a specific number of carb grams for two or three days—say, 30 to 40 grams—and then measure your ketones on each of those days to get an average.

  Then choose a different carb threshold, such as 40 grams, for two or three days and test again. The feedback you get will help you customize KetoFasting to your own body. This customization is an essential component of the program. Your carb threshold is dynamic, so periodically performing this testing will help you adapt your intake to meet your body's changing needs.

- **When you make substantial changes in your food choices.** Once you achieve fat burning and have maintained it for a few weeks to a month, you really only need to check your ketone levels if you make changes to your diet—for example, in response to a stressful event, a change in routine, or a long period of travel. At those times, you want to be sure that you are still burning plenty of fat for fuel.

  Test once a day until you are certain that your ketone levels have returned to their previous range. Your ultimate goal is achieving the metabolic flexibility you had as a healthy child! Kids go very easily into ketosis even when they eat large amounts of net carbs. By the time you reach adulthood, you have likely been following a high-carb diet for decades and your body has lost its ability to easily switch into fat-burning mode. By adopting KetoFast, you can gain that metabolic flexibility back.

- **As a way to monitor your long-term progress.** Ideally, you would check your ketone levels once or twice a week over the long term, choosing different times of the day to get the feedback and motivation you need to keep going.

Supplies You'll Need for This Phase

In addition to a ketone-measuring device (and its accompanying test strips, if necessary), it will also benefit you to pick up just a few more items to help you implement your KetoFast plan with accuracy and control.

- **Lancets and a lancet-holding device.** If you choose a blood ketone-measuring device, you'll also need lancets and a lancet-holding device in order to draw a drop of blood. Lancets are around $5 for a box of 100, and the devices are well under $10. There is no major difference that I am aware of between brands, so merely obtain and use whatever ones are convenient for you.

- **A digital food scale.** As I'll cover a little later in this chapter, an integral part of KetoFasting is using a tool that allows you to track your food intake. When you do this, it is advisable to use weight measurements (in grams), especially for small amounts. The most common mistake people make is to guess at the amounts of the foods they eat and enter those guesses into the food diary.

  For example, rather than estimating a tablespoon of seeds as one-half ounce, you need to weigh them on a scale. I made this mistake when I first embarked on KetoFasting. Once I realized my tallies were off and started weighing instead of just measuring my seeds, I found a tablespoon of psyllium was only 4 grams, while a tablespoon of cacao nibs weighed nearly three times that, at 11 grams.

  So if you don't already have an electronic digital kitchen food scale, plan on purchasing one soon. Prices start at under $20. Make sure to purchase one that measures up to a few pounds or kilos. These are usually accurate to 1 gram. If you need more precision, you can purchase scales that are accurate to 0.1

gram for about the same cost. Just be sure that they will still weigh a large quantity.

All digital scales have a tare function, also known as autozero. When you place the container on the scale and press tare, it resets the weight to zero. That way, you are only measuring the weight of the food and not the plate or container. Then just place the food you need to weigh into the container or onto the plate and enter that weight in grams into Cronometer.com/mercola (the online tool I recommend to track your food intake and give you invaluable feedback on how well you're feeding your body—more details on this in just a moment).

- **Measuring spoons.** You will want to have a set or two of stainless-steel measuring spoons so you can accurately measure out the food you then weigh on your digital scale.

Track Your Food Intake on Cronometer.com/mercola

From my perspective it is absolutely imperative that you use Cronometer, an online nutrient tracker, if you are going to have any hope of successfully implementing this program. Without an accurate analytical tool for tracking food intake, it will be virtually impossible to assess and fine-tune your program. Flying blind simply will not provide you with a comprehensive understanding of what you are actually eating, either in terms of calories or nutrients.

More important, you won't be able to determine the balance of macronutrients that's best for you; you won't know, for instance, how many grams of protein keep you in the fat-burning zone if you don't know how many grams of protein you eat.

Entering the foods you eat into Cronometer will allow you to keep an accurate record of everything you eat or drink. You can then combine this nutrient information with the biometric data that you collect—such as your weight and ketone levels—so you can understand how the foods you choose to eat are affecting your biochemistry and metabolism.

Cronometer.com/mercola is a free online service with four major advantages:

- **Data accuracy.** Cronometer is committed to using only high-quality macro- and micronutrient data obtained from the USDA National Nutrient Database and the Nutrition Coordinating Center Food and Nutrient Database.

  One note of caution: Cronometer has added commercial food products to its databases, but these entries are limited to the nutrition details listed on the label, which will not include many of the micronutrients that are important to your health.

  For example, Brazil nuts are an excellent source of selenium. But if you enter "Trader Joe's Brazil Nuts," you will not see how much selenium you're taking in as it's not listed on the nutrition label. You're better off entering the generic "Brazil nuts" from the USDA, which provides data on all the known nutrients for Brazil nuts. The same goes for the bar code scanner in the mobile app; these items contain only the label nutrition facts. So while it's very convenient to be able to log items with a bar code scanner, I only recommend doing so if you can't find an equivalent food from the higher-quality data sources. All items in the database contain macronutrient information so you can see at a glance how many grams of carb, protein, and fat you're taking in.

- **Elegant, easy-to-use graphical interface.** The real power of this program comes from the detailed graphs that show you exactly how close you come to meeting your personalized nutrient goals, down to the individual amino acids, vitamins, and minerals.

  You can tell Cronometer to set a dynamic macronutrient target for you that lines up with KetoFasting by choosing the "High Fat/Ketogenic" option in the pop-up box that opens when you click on "Calories Summary." When you do that, you will see a colored bar in the center of your dashboard that displays at a glance both the grams and the percentage of each macronutrient you consumed that day.

Many of the metrics in your dashboard also unveil further detail in pop-up displays if you hover your mouse over them. For example, you can mouse over the "Fat" bar and it will show you the precise percentage of monounsaturated, polyunsaturated, and saturated fats. Or, you can mouse over any other nutrient meter (such as carbs or fiber) and it will show you the top 10 foods in that category so you aren't just guessing about your intake. This is a convenient way to quickly identify the foods that are contributing to your nonfiber carbohydrates and protein totals for the day.

- **Allows you to keep a visual record of your progress.** Via a feature called "Snapshots," you can upload body fat percentage photos of yourself at different times during your KetoFasting journey and see the changes that occur in your physical appearance.

How to Use Cronometer for Cyclical Ketosis

To start, you can enter each food you eat separately, recording how much you ate in grams. It is important to actually measure here using a digital kitchen scale as mentioned above and not just guess. Remember, the accuracy of your analysis will only be as valid as the data you enter.

Later on, when you have some favorite go-to meals, you can enter them as your own personal recipes. You can also enter favorite recipes that you create on your own or find online or in keto cookbooks. Having your go-to meals already entered will make recording your daily intake quick and easy.

I suggest that each morning you enter all the foods you plan to eat that day, using it like a planner. This gives you the opportunity to view that day's analysis at the front end, *before* you eat it. It also gives you the flexibility to add or delete foods or change portion sizes to better reach your targets. This is far superior to entering the data after the fact, since you have lost the opportunity to make different choices that could have gotten you closer to your targets.

Along these lines, it is important to point out the obvious: You need to enter *every* bit of food or drink that passes your lips, even if you regret your choice as soon as you make it. Failing to track accurately and completely makes it virtually impossible to make sense of your data. Remember, the only person you hurt by not accurately recording what you eat is yourself.

Body Fat Percentage

How much fat you are carrying in your body is a vital gauge of your current metabolic health. Knowing your body fat percentage also allows you to calculate your lean body mass, which is essentially all parts of your body that aren't fat. Knowing your lean body mass will help you calculate precisely how much protein you should be eating on a daily basis, as well as how many calories you should consume on your KetoFast days.

Once you determine your body fat percentage, subtract it from 100 to determine your percentage of lean body tissue. From there, multiply that percentage by your current weight to get your total amount of lean body mass. For example, let's say that you use one or more of the methods I list below to learn that you have 30 percent body fat. That means you have 70 percent lean body tissue. Then you take 70 percent of your total body weight (multiply it by 0.7) to get your lean body mass. Finally, multiply your lean body mass in pounds by .5 to determine how many grams of protein you need to eat each day in order to maintain muscle mass. If you regularly eat more than this amount of protein a day, your body will tend to convert the excess protein into glucose, meaning that eating too much protein can knock you out of ketosis and can contribute to excess fat stores.

There are several ways to determine how much body fat you are carrying. Each has its pluses and minuses. I've listed them below in order of cost, complexity, and accuracy, from lowest to highest:

- **Photo approximation.** The easiest and least expensive way to gauge your body fat percentage is to take a photo of yourself in your underwear and then compare it to photos of people at different body fat percentages. You can find the photos for comparison on Cronometer.com/mercola or by doing an Internet search for "body fat percentage" and selecting the "Images" tab on the results page. This is obviously not the most accurate method, but it can give you a very loose estimation of where you might be and what the next stage in personal health actually looks like.

- **Skin calipers.** This low-tech method involves using an inexpensive, lightweight handheld device known as a skin caliper to measure the thickness of a fold of your skin and the fat that lies beneath it. Your doctor or skilled personal trainer can measure you, or if you want the flexibility of doing it yourself, calipers cost anywhere from a couple of dollars to a couple of hundred dollars and resemble a small pair of tongs. They can measure distance down to a millimeter. They can readily be purchased on Amazon and come with comprehensive instructions and formulas that will calculate your body fat percentage.

  Although there is always the possibility of error, calipers are one of the most time-tested and accurate ways to measure body fat. For results to be truly helpful, it's best to engage the help of another person—particularly for women, who need to measure the skin fold on the back of the upper arm, a difficult-to-reach area—and to use that same person to take your measurements each time. You'll also need to either perform some simple calculations on your own or use an online calculator developed for just this purpose to translate those measurements into your body fat percentage.

- **Digital scale with body fat readings.** This approach can be as simple as stepping on a specific type of scale that measures body fat, readily available online starting at about $25. These scales use bioelectrical impedance analysis (BIA), which sends an electrical signal through your body, where it will pass easily through lean body mass—which is up to 75 percent water, a good conductor of electricity—but be impeded by your fat tissue, which contains low amounts of water. This measurement, along with other factors—such as your height, weight, age, and sex, which you enter into the device—is then used to calculate your percentage of body fat, lean body mass, and other body composition measurements.

  While this analysis is certainly convenient, there is some concern that it may not be as accurate in nutritional ketosis because making the switch to fat burning has a diuretic effect. This is because every molecule of glycogen is stored with 3 to 4 grams of water, so when you burn through your glycogen stores on your way to fat burning, you also release water weight and this may throw off the accuracy of BIA.

  Although the absolute value may be off a bit, a BIA scale is relatively accurate and typically very consistent. Even though the number itself might not be correct, it will accurately measure your body fat day-to-day variability, which is a far more reliable monitor than your body weight.

- **Dual-energy X-ray absorptiometry (DEXA) scan.** A DEXA scan is an X-ray that gives a detailed reading of overall and regional fat mass, lean mass, and bone mass; you may be familiar with it, particularly if you are a woman, as this method is frequently used to measure bone density. Although it is considered by many to be very accurate in measuring body fat, Dr. Jason Fung finds that it falsely measures lean body mass. The use of X-rays makes the DEXA scan one of the most expensive methods, as well as a source of exposure to radiation, although at very minor levels. You'll likely have to do a little digging to find a place to have the scan done—many hospitals, universities with exercise physiology centers, and health-care facilities have one—and then you'll have to pay anywhere from $50 to $150 or more for the scan. Keep in mind that for a DEXA scan to be truly helpful, you'll need to repeat it in a few months to see how your body composition has changed. (Make it very clear when you make your appointment that you want to test for lean body mass, not bone density.)

General Body Fat Percentage Guidelines from the American Council on Exercise

Classification	Women (% fat)	Men (% fat)
Essential Fat	10–13%	2–5%
Athletes	14–20%	6–13%
Fitness	21–24%	14–17%
Acceptable	25–31%	18–24%
Obese	32% and higher	25% and higher

Three of the Safest Sugar Alternatives

1. **Lo han (lo han kuo) or monk fruit** is my absolute favorite natural sweetener. It is similar to stevia, and is a bit more expensive, but I think it tastes much better. I use the vanilla Lakanto brand, which is available on Amazon. In China, the lo han fruit has

been used as a sweetener for centuries, and it's about 200 times sweeter than sugar. It received FDA GRAS (generally regarded as safe) status in 2009.

2.   **Stevia** is a highly sweet herb derived from the leaf of the South American stevia plant. It is sold as a liquid and as a powder and is completely safe in its natural form. It can be used to sweeten most dishes and drinks, although be careful with it—because it's so sweet, a little goes a long way. Keep in mind that the same cannot be said for some brands that make use of only certain active ingredients of stevia and not the entire plant. Usually it's the *synergistic* effect of all the agents in the plant that provides the overall health effect, which oftentimes includes built-in protection against potentially damaging effects.

3.   **Sugar alcohols** have "ol" at the end of their name— these include erythritol, xylitol, sorbitol, maltitol, mannitol, and glycerol. They're not as sweet as sugar, and they do contain fewer calories, but they're not calorie free.

Step Four: Add in One to Two Days of "Feasting" Each Week

As beneficial as it is to achieve the metabolic flexibility to be able to burn fat, once you start producing more than 0.5 mmol/L of ketones, you need to start cycling in one or two days a week of higher net carbs. On these days, you can eat between 100 and 150 grams of net carbs, as opposed to the 20 to 50 grams you want to eat on your ketogenic days.

You don't want to stay on a ketogenic diet for the long term. One of the biggest downsides is that the high-net carbs such as vegetables and fruits that have large amounts of resistant starch (fiber) are a source of food for your beneficial gut bacteria; depriving yourself of these foods will negatively impact your microbiome.

Step Five: Add in One Day of KetoFasting Each Week

Remember that you will not start KetoFasting until you have been able to flip your metabolic switch and burn fat for fuel as demonstrated by your ability to generate ketones (over 0.5 mmol/L). On these days when you only consume a very limited amount of calories, you will virtually deplete all of your stored glycogen and facilitate lipolysis and release of fat-soluble toxins.

You can start KetoFasting once a week for the first month, and if you are doing well with that, you can progress to two days a week of KetoFasting. If you are facing obesity or a disease challenge, then I advise you to work as quickly as you can to KetoFasting up to twice a week. The other days you should be doing a cyclical ketogenic diet. **Your eating strategy should include three to four days of eating a ketogenic diet, one to two days of eating a higher level of net carbs, and one to two days of KetoFasting, depending on what feels right to your body.**

You can continue your twice-a-week KetoFasting until you reach your health goals and/or optimize your weight. At that point you can reduce your frequency to a few times a month to help your body eliminate all the toxins you are regularly exposed to and also to help combat the aging process by activating stem cells and autophagy.

Calculate Your KetoFast Calorie Target and Breakdown

To determine how many calories you should have on your KetoFast days, you need to multiply your lean body mass in pounds by 3.5. You should arrive at a number somewhere between 300 and 600 calories (300 calories is typical for a small woman and 600 calories for a larger man).

On your fasting days you will want to keep your carbohydrates below 20 grams. Below 10 grams would be even better, as this will make it easier for you to enter ketosis. The reason for this is it typically takes at least a full 24 to 36 hours to deplete the glycogen stores in your liver. The 18-hour daily intermittent fast will not fully exhaust the sugar stored in your liver. But when you go the next 24 hours with only 10 to 20 grams of carbs, combined with a low amount of calories, your liver glycogen will become exhausted and you will trigger the metabolic magic of autophagy.

Initially I thought that it would be best to also limit your protein intake based on traditional fasting recommendations. However, I tested this for several months and found that for me, it was best to decrease my regular protein intake only by half. In my case my daily non-fasting protein intake is 80 to 100 grams, so I take about 45 to 50 grams on the partial fast days. It's likely to be the same for you.

I found when I changed this strategy I would not lose as much lean body mass. When I restricted protein to 20 grams or even lower, I would lose 7 pounds after my partial fast. After I more than doubled the protein, the weight loss decreased to only 3 pounds and my blood sugar and ketone levels remained high.

However, I would not increase proteins that have high amounts of branched chain amino acids, like whey protein and red meat, as they would activate mTOR and inhibit autophagy. Collagen protein would be an excellent choice to use during these days, as it is very low in branched chain amino acids and will conserve your connective tissue.

A plant-based vegan chocolate protein powder would also be a good option. We have one on our site that tastes great and is low in these amino acids. These are the two primary proteins I use on my partial fasting days, in addition to 15 grams of fermented chlorella.

In my mind this is a better strategy if you are older than 65 and normal body weight, as it should preserve your lean body mass better, which is vital to stay healthy as you age.

So after you add all the foods you choose for partial fasting, this will provide a certain number of calories. Since you know the number of calories you need as per the calculation above, all you need to do is add the remaining calories as fat, preferably in the form of coconut, MCT, or even better, caprylic acid (C8) MCT oil (described below in more detail). This should result in 65 to 85 percent of your calories coming from fat and will dramatically increase ketones generated during your fast. Ideally it would be best to have all these calories as one meal rather than breaking them up throughout the day.

Here is the important part, though: Note the time you finish your meal and don't eat again for another 24 hours. So you will be going into the 24-hour fast with an 18-hour intermittent fast, which will give you nearly 48 hours of partial fasting. Most people find it easiest to maintain this 24-hour fast by having their last meal in the late morning.

Choose Your Recipes Well for KetoFast

Cronometer comes in even handier on your KetoFast days, since you have an even tighter window of total calories and macronutrient ratios. In order to reap the maximum benefits of being in a fasted state, accuracy is highly important on your fasting days. You will have to be careful to precisely measure your food with a digital kitchen scale. If you are just guessing, you could sabotage the effectiveness of your KetoFast program.

It is crucial that the foods you eat on these fasting days be organic, because you don't want to subject yourself to any additional toxins at a time when your body will be busily liberating stored toxins from your fat cells. Cruciferous vegetables will be especially helpful as they are loaded with phytonutrients that will support your detoxification process.

If you are like most people, it would be far easier for you to implement this program if someone did the work for you. And that is precisely what I did. The companion to this book, *KetoFast Cookbook*, is written with Australian celebrity chef Pete Evans, who has put together more than 40 delicious recipes that are appropriate for your fasting days.

But it gets even better. All the recipes are already entered into Cronometer, so you don't need to enter any foods. You merely type in the recipe you need after you have clicked on the "Add Foods" tab. Then all you need to do is add enough coconut or C8 MCT oil to the recipe to meet your calorie target. For most people this will be one to two tablespoons. Alternatively, if you are drinking black coffee or tea, you could add the coconut or MCT oil to those.

Coconut and MCT Oil

Coconut oil has been a dietary and beauty staple for millennia. It fights all kinds of microbes, from viruses to bacteria to protozoa, many of which can be harmful, and is a fabulous source of high-quality fat. Around 50 percent of the fat in coconut oil is lauric acid, which is rarely found in nature. In fact, coconut oil has a greater proportion of lauric acid than any other food. Your body converts lauric acid into monolaurin, a monoglyceride (a single fat attached to a glycerol molecule, unlike three fats which would be a triglyceride) that can actually destroy many lipid-coated viruses such as HIV, herpes, influenza, measles, gram-negative bacteria, and protozoa such as *Giardia lamblia*.

MCT oil is coconut oil's more concentrated cousin. Most commercially available MCT consists of equal amounts of caprylic acid (C8, a fatty acid with eight carbon atoms in its molecular structure) and capric acid (C10, a 10-carbon fatty acid).

Normally when you eat a fatty food it is broken down in the small intestine through the action of bile salts and lipase, a pancreatic enzyme. But medium-chain triglycerides (MCT) are able to bypass this process; they diffuse across the intestinal membrane and go directly to your liver via the hepatic portal.

Once there, especially if you are in nutritional ketosis—burning fat for fuel—they are quickly converted into ketones, which are then released back into your bloodstream and transported throughout your body, including to your brain, to be used as clean-burning fuel.

For this reason, MCT oil is a great way to take in some extra fat, as it is odorless and tasteless and is therefore easy to consume straight off the spoon. Its rapid conversion to energy can help you stay on the KetoFast plan in those moments when your hunger is high and appropriate food is scarce.

The only hitch is that this efficiency does come with a small cost. Your liver may not be able to process that much fat quickly, so it may dump some of it back into your intestines, where it can cause stomach upset and very loose stools if you consume too much. You can consume MCT oil every day, but you must start slowly and build up your dosage over time so you can increase your tolerance to it.

Start with one teaspoon once a day, preferably combined with food, and if you don't experience loose stools or other GI symptoms, gradually work your way up. Some people use up to a tablespoon or two with each meal, but most only need a tablespoon or two per day. If at any point you develop digestive upset or loose stools, go back to your previous dose and stay there for a few days. Increasing your fiber intake can also help ward off MCT oil–induced diarrhea and bloating.

My personal preference for MCT oil, even though it is more expensive, is straight C8 (caprylic acid), as it converts to ketones far more rapidly and efficiently than other versions of MCT oil, most of which contain close to a 50:50 combination of C8 and C10 (capric acid) fats. It may be easier on your digestion as well. The other reason I prefer C8 MCT oil is that it will convert to ketones far more effectively, and increased ketones have many health benefits, especially when you are partial fasting.

Whatever MCT oil you buy, it is just as important to make sure that it is hexane- and chemical-free as it is when purchasing coconut oil; you don't want to add to your toxic load, especially when you are burning fat for fuel and thus liberating fat-stored toxins into the bloodstream. And be sure to store it away from sunlight in an opaque bottle that limits light exposure. Although MCT is not usually used as a cooking oil, you can use it in some recipes; just avoid heating it over 320 degrees. For example, you can substitute it for part of the oil that you would use to make mayonnaise or a salad dressing, blend it with vegetables to make a sauce, or add it to smoothies or soups. You can also add it to coffee or tea along with another fat like ghee; blend it well and enjoy it for an energy boost.

There's just one thing to keep in mind: Because MCT oil is so readily converted to fuel, and that fuel can be utilized by your brain and heart, if you take it at night, you may be too hyperalert to sleep. That said, if you are following the KetoFast program, you will be avoiding all food for a minimum of three hours before sleep, so this should not be an issue.

Caution: Individuals with liver cancer, elevated liver enzymes, extensive liver metastases, or liver disease *should not* use MCT oil. However, they can still use coconut oil, because it doesn't create ketones as readily as MCT oil.

Can You Exercise During KetoFast?

It would be best to avoid any strenuous exercise on the days you are KetoFasting. These are not the days when you want to do high-intensity exercises or strength training. Think of them as rest and repair days. You should move regularly throughout the day, and limited walking is fine, but try to limit your steps to less than 5,000 to 7,000 on days you're partially fasting. Ideally, you would also use a near-infrared sauna to facilitate the cellular detoxification process and excretion of toxins through sweating.

SUPPLEMENTS TO SUPPORT YOUR DETOXIFICATION

The following supplements will help your body complete the detoxification process and minimize any damaging effects from the toxins that may get liberated from your fat stores.

Nutrients

- **Ubiquinol (better reduced form of CoQ10): 100 to 150 milligrams twice a day.** Coenzyme Q is necessary for your mitochondrial energy production and regulates the expression of genes that are important for inflammatory processes, growth, and detoxification reactions.[10]

- **Organic psyllium: one to two tablespoons.** Psyllium, a soluble fiber that will help you move the toxins out of your body, contains about 18 calories per tablespoon, so be sure to add this into your Cronometer data to hit your appropriate calorie target.

- **High-quality probiotic.** Follow the dosage guidelines on the package. Look for one with *L. rhamnosus*, which has been shown to reduce pesticide toxicity,[11] and *L. plantarum*, which has been shown to reduce the negative effects of mycotoxin exposure.[12] My Complete Probiotics provide an excellent source of these and other useful strains, but there are other companies that sell probiotics that contain these strains; just make sure that they are high potency.

- **Phosphatidylcholine.** This is a special type of fat called a phospholipid that has a phosphate group and choline molecule attached to it. It is found in every single cell of your body and it makes up more than half of your cell membranes.

  Phosphatidylcholine can help displace the toxins that are embedded in your cell membranes. Choline contains three methyl groups, making it one of your body's major methyl donors to contribute to the methylation pathway necessary for detoxification. In fact, 60 percent of your body's methyl groups come from choline.

  In addition to rebuilding cell membranes, phosphatidylcholine helps your body eliminate toxins. It supports liver function (and is in fact a treatment for fatty liver disease), and assists with dumping waste out of your cells. By supporting cellular function and your liver, you can more easily eliminate toxins when you are regularly using phosphatidyl choline. The dose would be about 1 to 2 grams and liposomal preparations are preferred.

- **Bitters.** Bitters have been used medicinally since ancient times for digestive ailments and were developed as patent medicines in the 1800s (typically marketed as tonics). The term *bitters* traditionally refers to alcohol-based extracts of the bark, leaves, roots, or flowers of bitter-tasting plants.

The bitter taste passes through one of your cranial nerves to a special group of cells in your brain. The taste is interpreted there as bitter, and causes a stimulation of your vagus nerve to both the salivary gland and the stomach to increase the secretion of bile.[13] This is important because your bile will contain the toxins that have been liberated by KetoFasting and you will want to make sure they are eliminated into your colon and ultimately your stool.

The bitter formula I use is a liposomal preparation that has phosphatidylcholine and is called Dr. Shade's Liver Sauce™, made by Quicksilver Scientific. A typical dose would be one tablespoon held under the tongue for 30 seconds. Urban Moonshine is a lower-cost organic bitter formula that can be used. Alternatively, you can create your own formula with some of the following bitters:

- **Gentian.** This herb offers the long-known action of bitters, which increase the secretion of gastric juice and bile due to the stimulation of gustatory nerves in the mouth.[14]

- **Dandelion.** Dandelion has acute anti-inflammatory activities and protects against cholecystokinin (a bile-moving enzyme) and pancreatitis.[15] Pharmaceutical compounds that have been identified in dandelion extract include phenolic acids and flavonoids.[16, 17] Studies have shown that some of these compounds have therapeutic effects in inflammation.[18, 19] Dandelion also contains triterpenes and sterols, which are inhibitors of inflammation.[20]

- **Solidago (goldenrod).** Solidago, commonly known as goldenrod, is widely hailed for its beneficial actions on the urinary tract. It is rich in flavonoids, some of which have been shown to activate enzymes that play a crucial role in detoxification.[21]

- **Myrrh.** This tree resin native to the Middle East is hailed for its antioxidant properties; animal testing has found that it can help protect the liver from damage due to lead exposure.[22]

BINDERS

If you don't consume binders when you're fasting, you run the risk of retoxifying your body and exposing yourself to more damage from the toxins you've unleashed from the safe cocoons of your fat cells. A binder does just what it sounds like it should do: It binds with substances in the GI tract so that those substances can be excreted through the feces.

There are a large number of binders on the market. I am recommending the ones below based on my review of the literature and personal experience.[23] It is important to know that all binders need to be taken on an empty stomach, either one hour before or two hours after a meal. If you don't do this, the binders will actually bind the nutrients in your food and make them unavailable and useless.

- **Activated charcoal: 5 to 6 grams.** Activated charcoal is well known to remove toxins from water and is the primary filtration mechanism for most home water filter systems because it is so effective at removing chlorine, disinfection by-products, and drugs that are in the water supply. Like chitosan and modified citrus pectin, it is not magic and needs to be timed appropriately.

  If you take it with food it will bind the nutrients in your food, which is not what you want. But taken at the appropriate time in the detox process—i.e., during your fast—it will serve to eliminate the toxins that the liver is passing into the bile and subsequently into the colon, where the charcoal can effectively bind to them and eliminate them in your stool. It has been used to remove lead[24] and to treat iron over-dose[25] and mercury poisoning.[26]

- **Chitosan: 2 to 3 grams.** Chitosan is a derivative of chitin, which is a naturally fibrous material found in the exoskeletons of crustaceans and insects.[27] It has been shown to be useful in removing heavy metals[28, 29, 30] and even radionuclides.[31]

- **Modified citrus pectin: 5 grams, one to three times a day.** Pectin, a complex carbohydrate (polysaccharide) found in virtually all plants, helps to bind cells together and provides a structural framework for maintaining the shape and integrity of cell membranes. A modified form of citrus pectin derived from the pulp and peel of citrus fruits has been shown to attach to cancer cells to prevent them from spreading throughout the body, pointing the way to a potentially safe approach for preventing or reducing cancer metastases.[32] It is also very effective for binding heavy metals.[33, 34]

- **Chlorella: 5 to 15 grams.** Chlorella, single-celled fresh-water algae, is often referred to as a near-perfect food because it supplies a rich source of amino acids, essential fatty acids, vitamins, and minerals. Because chlorella can be considered a food, it should not be used on your partial fast days as it will give you too many calories and proteins.

    Algae and other aquatic plants possess the capacity to take up toxic trace metals from their environment, resulting in an internal concentration greater than those of the surrounding waters. This property has been exploited as a mean for treating industrial effluent containing metals before they are discharged and to recover the bioavailable fraction of the metal.

    It is best to use broken cell wall chlorella because its cell wall is difficult to digest. It is also wise to chew the chlorella to improve its absorption and action. It has been reported to suppress methylmercury transfer to the fetus in pregnant mice.[35] Even though it will help bind mercury and other heavy metals, it has a significant amount of protein, so you do not want to take it with your other binders, but still take it one hour before or two hours after your meal.[36]

One exception: If you choose to eat seafood that might be contaminated with mercury, it would be wise to eat it with a large dose of chlorella, which will tend to bind the mercury and prevent it from being absorbed. It is best to start slow with chlorella to make sure you don't have a reaction to it. Try ½ to 1 gram at first, adding ½ to 1 gram per day until you have obtained your target dose.

Take chlorella on your non-KetoFast days as it contains a fair amount of protein. If you do choose to use 15 grams of chlorella on your KetoFast days, you will need to add 10 grams of protein to your Cronometer data, which would quite possibly exceed your protein needs for the day.

LIQUIDS ACCEPTABLE FOR KETOFAST DAYS

- Water, unlimited
- Tea, unlimited (but choose from the ones below)
- Coffee (no cream), up to six cups a day, hot or iced, must be organic
- Homemade broth, as long as you maintain your calories in the target range

Healthy Detox Teas

- Rooibos and honeybush (a cousin of rooibos) are traditional South African herbal beverages rich in unique polyphenolic antioxidants. They can improve glutathione redox status[37] and your ability to convert fat-soluble toxins to water-soluble ones so they can be eliminated.

- Dandelion root is commonly used in traditional Chinese medicine and has been shown to reduce swelling and inflammation and aid in detoxification.[38]

- Chamomile for nighttime. It will help you sleep better, and it also has about one percent apigenin, which has the additional benefit of inhibiting the CD38 enzyme that is the highest extracellular consumer of NAD+, so this will increase your NAD+ levels, which are very beneficial for detoxification.[39]

What You Can Add to Your Water

- Any of the accepted natural sweeteners that are described on pages 127–128.

- Lime slices (don't consume the limes or any other fruits)

- Lemon slices

- Apple cider vinegar that is raw, organic, and contains "the mother," or the culture of beneficial bacteria that converted regular apple cider into vinegar

- Healthy salt such as Celtic, Redmond, or Himalayan

What You Can Add to Your Coffee or Tea (Up to One Tablespoon):

- Any of the accepted natural sweeteners that are described on page 127–128

- Coconut oil (hexane- and chemical-free)

- C8 MCT oil

- Butter (organic, pastured, preferably raw)

- Ghee (organic)

- Heavy cream (organic, pastured, preferably raw)

- Ground cinnamon

- Lemon (for tea)

WHAT YOU CAN DO
IF YOU ARE FEELING HUNGRY

Psyllium husk is a soluble fiber best known for its ability to treat constipation and is the active ingredient in Metamucil. It grows around the world but is most commonly found in India, which remains the largest producer of psyllium husk today. The whole seed has been used in traditional Iranian medicine for hundreds of years.

The outer coat (the husk) is ground down into *mucilage*, a clear, colorless, gelatinous dietary fiber that confers the majority of health benefits in both humans and animals. Psyllium fiber beneficially impacts colon function and has been shown to regulate the intestinal barrier and decrease proinflammatory cytokines and decreased tight junction protein expression in the colon.[40]

The interesting characteristic of psyllium husk is that it is loaded with soluble fibers; even though a tablespoon has 18 calories, they are all digestive-resistant carbs, so it adds zero carbs to your dietary targets. You can put a tablespoon in a glass of water and let it form a gel and eat it like a porridge. It will fill your stomach, alleviating your hunger pangs.

However, it is very important to understand that most of psyllium, especially in brand products like Metamucil, is not organic and could be loaded with pesticides. So if you are going to use psyllium, it is absolutely imperative that you make sure it is organic, otherwise you will merely be reintroducing additional toxins into your body.

You could also use the Pure Power Organic Mitomix Seed Blend, available on my website, that is a mixture of flax seeds, whole psyllium husks, chia seeds, black sesame, and cumin seeds. One tablespoon of this mixture has about the same amount of calories as psyllium husk alone but has an additional 2 grams of protein. You can also let this seed mixture soak for a while and eat it with a spoon.

HOW TO KETOFAST

1 Compress your eating window to 6-8 hours for one month.

2 Determine your total calorie intake for KetoFast days by multiplying your lean body mass x 3.5. For most this is between 300-600 calories.

3 Determine your grams of protein by cutting your normal daily intake by half. Determine calories from protein by multiplying protein grams x 4.

4 Keep total carb under 20 grams, 10 would be even better. Determine calories from carbs by multiplying carb grams x 4.

5 Add protein and carb calories and subtract from your total calorie intake for the day.

6 This number is the number of fat calories you need. You can divide by 9 to obtain the number of fat grams for your recipe.

7 Create your one meal recipe for the day which should ideally be your breakfast.

8 Entire above process is highly simplified if you use Cronometer as they have set up their software to easily make these calculations for you. Additionally, recipes for KetoFast Cookbook are pre entered.

CHAPTER 9

MONITOR YOUR PROGRESS WITH THESE LAB TESTS

How can you tell if your efforts to improve your health and detox your body are working? First, consider the subjective things you experience as a result of upgrading your diet and incorporating KetoFasting into your regular routine: things like sleeping better, losing weight, and having more energy.

It's also helpful to see quantitative evidence that your hard work is paying off. For that, there are eight health-screening tests I suggest you take as you embark on your KetoFast plan, and again at least three months in. It's so gratifying to see your markers of health improve; it also encourages you to keep going.

While studies suggest the health of Americans suffers due to excessive, unnecessary, and/or ineffective medical tests and treatments, certain lab tests can offer truly important clues about your health. Unfortunately, some of the most valuable tests are rarely ordered by conventional physicians. What's more, even if your doctor does order some or all of these tests, the ranges that are considered "normal" are not necessarily ideal for optimal health.

So which lab tests should you look to as a gauge of your health, and what are the ideal reference ranges you're looking for? Here are the eight tests I recommend for everyone who wants to take control of their health.

NO. 1—VITAMIN D

Optimizing your vitamin D is one of the easiest and least-expensive things you can do for your health. My recommendation is to get your vitamin D level tested twice a year, when your level is likely to be at its lowest (midwinter) and highest (midsummer).

This is particularly important if you're pregnant or planning a pregnancy, or if you have cancer. Based on the research done and data collected by GrassrootsHealth (grassrootshealth. net), a nonprofit public health organization dedicated to sharing research on vitamin D with practitioners and the public, 40 ng/mL (100 nm/L) is the cutoff point for sufficiency to prevent a wide range of diseases. For example, most cancers occur in people with a vitamin D blood level between 10 and 40 ng/mL,[1, 2] and published data suggests a whopping 80 percent of breast cancer recurrences—four out of five—could be prevented simply by optimizing vitamin D and nothing else.[3, 4]

For optimal health and disease prevention, a level between 60 and 80 ng/mL (150 to 200 nm/L) appears to be ideal.[5] While the American Medical Association claims 20 ng/mL is sufficient, research suggests 20 ng/mL is barely adequate for the prevention of osteomalacia (softening of the bones), and clearly far too low for other disease prevention or improvement.

When it comes to dosage, you need to take whatever dose required to get you into the optimal range, with 40 ng/mL being the low-end cutoff for sufficiency. Research[6] suggests it would require 9,600 IUs of vitamin D per day to get 97.5 percent of the population to reach 40 ng/mL, but there's a wide variance in individual requirements.

If you've been getting regular sun exposure; have eaten vitamin D–rich foods such as beef liver, mushrooms, and organic free-range egg yolks;[7] and/or taken a certain amount of vitamin D_3 for a number of months and retesting reveals you're still not within the recommended range, then you know you need to increase your dosage.

Over time, with continued testing, you'll find your individual sweet spot and have a good idea of how much you need to take to maintain a year-round level of 60 to 80 ng/mL. GrassrootsHealth offers vitamin D testing at a great value through its D*action study, and has an online vitamin D calculator you can use to estimate your vitamin D_3 dosage once you know your current serum level.

NO. 2—RBC MAGNESIUM

Magnesium deficiency is extremely common, and recent research[8] shows even subclinical deficiency can jeopardize your heart health. Magnesium is important for brain health, detoxification, cellular health and function, energy production,[9, 10] regulation of insulin sensitivity,[11] normal cell division,[12] the optimization of your mitochondria,[13] and much more.

Magnesium resides at the center of the chlorophyll molecule, so if you rarely eat fresh leafy greens, you're probably not getting much magnesium from your diet. Furthermore, while eating organic whole foods[14] will help optimize your magnesium intake, it's still not a surefire way to ward off magnesium deficiency, as most soils have become severely depleted of nutrients, including magnesium.

Magnesium absorption is also dependent on having sufficient amounts of selenium, parathyroid hormone, and vitamins B_6 and D, and is hindered by excess ethanol, salt, coffee, and phosphoric acid in soda. Sweating, stress, lack of sleep, excessive menstruation, and certain drugs (especially diuretics and proton-pump inhibitors) also deplete your body of magnesium.[15]

For these reasons, many experts recommend taking supplemental magnesium. The recommended dietary allowance for magnesium is 310 to 420 milligrams per day depending on your age and sex,[16] but many experts believe you may need 600 to 900 milligrams per day, which is more in line with the magnesium uptake during the Paleolithic period.[17] Personally, I believe many may benefit from amounts as high as 1 to 2 grams (1,000 to 2,000 milligrams) of elemental magnesium per day in divided doses.

The key to effectively using these higher doses, however, is to make sure you avoid loose bowel movements, as that will disrupt your gut microbiome, which would be highly counterproductive. One of the best ways to up your magnesium intake is with magnesium threonate, as it appears to be the most efficient at penetrating cell membranes, including your mitochondria and blood-brain barrier. Another effective way to boost your magnesium level is to take Epsom salt (magnesium sulfate) baths, as the magnesium effectively absorbs through your skin.

I prepare a supersaturated solution of Epsom salts by dissolving seven tablespoons of the salt into six ounces of water and heating it until all the salt has dissolved. I pour it into a dropper bottle and then apply it to my skin and rub fresh aloe leaves over it to dissolve it. This is an easy and inexpensive way to increase your magnesium and will allow you to get higher dosages into your body without having to deal with its laxative effects.

Optimizing your magnesium level is particularly important when taking supplemental vitamin D, as your body cannot properly utilize the vitamin if your magnesium level is insufficient.[18, 19] The reason for this is because magnesium is required for the actual activation of vitamin D.

If your magnesium level is too low, the vitamin D will simply get stored in its inactive form. As an added boon, when your magnesium level is sufficiently high, it will be far easier to optimize your vitamin D level, as you'll require a far lower dose.[20] In fact, research[21] shows higher magnesium intake helps reduce your risk of vitamin D deficiency—likely by activating more of it.

NO. 3—OMEGA-3 INDEX

Like vitamin D, your omega-3 level is also a powerful predictor of your all-cause mortality risk and plays a vital role in overall health, especially your heart and brain health.

Recent research[22] funded by the National Institutes of Health found that a higher omega-3 index was associated with a lower risk for cardiovascular events, coronary heart disease events, and strokes. Omega-3 also helps decrease pain, especially when combined with vitamin D.

(Omega-3 fats are precursors to mediators of inflammation called prostaglandins, which is, in part, how they help reduce pain. Anti-inflammatory painkillers also work by manipulating prostaglandins.)

The omega-3 index is a blood test that measures the amount of EPA and DHA omega-3 fatty acids in your red blood cell membranes. Your index is expressed as a percent of your total RBC fatty acids.

The omega-3 index reflects your tissue levels of EPA and DHA, and has been validated as a stable, long-term marker of your omega-3 status. An omega-3 index above 8 percent is associated with the lowest risk of death from heart disease. An index below 4 percent puts you at the highest risk of heart disease–related mortality. If you're below 8 percent, increase your omega-3 intake and retest in three to six months.

You can save money by getting the combined vitamin D and omega-3 index testing kit offered by GrassrootsHealth as part of its consumer-sponsored research.

Your best sources of animal-based omega-3 are small, cold-water fatty fish such as anchovies, herrings, and sardines. Wild Alaskan salmon is another good source that is low in mercury and other environmental toxins. These fish are also a decent source of vitamin D, making them even more beneficial.

If you're not eating these foods on a regular basis, you can add quality supplements of fish oil or krill oil to your diet. The latter is my preferred choice, as it contains DHA and EPA in a form that's less prone to oxidation. The fatty acids in krill oil are also bound to phospholipids, which allow the DHA and EPA to travel efficiently into your hepatic system so that they're more bioavailable. Studies[23] have shown that krill oil may be 48 times more potent than fish oil.

NO. 4—FASTING INSULIN

Insulin resistance is a driving factor for virtually all chronic disease, making fasting insulin testing a really important health screen. Any meal high in processed carbs typically generates a rapid rise in your blood glucose. To compensate, your pancreas secretes insulin into your bloodstream, which lowers your blood sugar.

If your body failed to produce insulin to do this, you would likely go into a hyperglycemic coma and die. Insulin, however, will also catalyze the conversion of excess sugar into fat cells.

Typically, the more insulin you make, the fatter you become. If you consistently consume a high-sugar, high-grain diet, your blood glucose level will be correspondingly high, and over time your body becomes desensitized to insulin, requiring more and more insulin to get the job done.

Eventually, you become insulin resistant and prone to weight gain, then prediabetes, and then full-blown diabetes. Prediabetes[24] is defined as an elevation in fasting blood glucose above 100 mg/dL but lower than 125 mg/dl, at which point it formally becomes type 2 diabetes.

However, any fasting blood sugar regularly above 90 mg/dL is really suggestive of insulin resistance, and the seminal work of Dr. Joseph Kraft suggests 80 percent—8 out of 10—Americans are in fact insulin resistant.[25] Although he recommends an oral glucose tolerance test that also measures insulin, this is a far more challenging test, and for most a fasting insulin test will suffice.

The fasting blood insulin test is far better than a fasting glucose test, as it reflects how healthy your blood glucose levels are over time. It's important to realize that it's possible to have low fasting glucose but still have a significantly elevated insulin level. And yes, it must be fasting for at least eight hours, otherwise the results are nearly meaningless.

A normal fasting blood insulin level is below five, but ideally, you'll want it below three. If your insulin level is higher than three, the most effective way to optimize it is to reduce or eliminate all forms of dietary sugar. Intermittent fasting, partial fasting, and/or water fasting are also effective, and intermittent fasting combined with a ketogenic diet appears to be the most aggressively effective of all.

NO. 5—SERUM FERRITIN

Ferritin is the major iron storage protein in your body, so the ferritin test is an indirect way to measure the iron stores in your body. For adults, I strongly recommend getting a serum ferritin test on an annual basis, as iron overload can be every bit as dangerous as vitamin D deficiency. While iron is necessary for biological function, when you get too much, it can do tremendous harm by increasing oxidative stress. Unfortunately, the first thing people think about when they hear "iron" is anemia, or iron deficiency, not realizing that iron overload is actually a more common problem, and far more dangerous.

When iron reacts with hydrogen peroxide, typically in your mitochondria, dangerous hydroxyl free radicals are formed. These are among the most damaging free radicals known. They are highly reactive and can damage DNA, cell membranes, and proteins. They contribute to mitochondrial dysfunction, which in turn is at the heart of most chronic degenerative diseases.

Virtually all adult men and postmenopausal women are at risk for iron overload since they do not shed blood on a regular basis. Humans are not at all designed to excrete excess iron, as it is simply stored for a rainy day when you might need it to recover from some type of trauma that has resulted in blood loss.

There's also an inherited disease, hemochromatosis, which causes your body to accumulate excessive and dangerous levels of iron. If left untreated, high iron can contribute to cancer, heart disease, diabetes, neurodegenerative diseases, and many other health problems, including gouty arthritis.[26]

As with many other lab tests, the "normal" range for serum ferritin is far from ideal.[27] A level of 200 to 300 ng/mL falls within the normal range for women and men respectively, but if you're in this range, know that you're virtually guaranteed to develop some sort of health problem.

An ideal level for adult men and nonmenstruating women is actually somewhere between 30 and 40 ng/mL. (You do not want to be below 20 ng/mL or much above 40 ng/mL.) The most commonly used threshold for iron deficiency in clinical studies is 12 to 15 ng/mL.[28]

You may also consider doing a gamma-glutamyl transpeptidase (GGT) test. GGT is a liver enzyme correlated with iron toxicity and all-cause mortality. Not only will the GGT test tell you if you have liver damage, it's also an excellent marker for excess free iron and a great indicator of your risk of sudden cardiac death.

In recent years, researchers have discovered GGT is highly interactive with iron, and when serum ferritin and GGT are both high, you are at significantly increased risk of chronic health problems, because then you have a combination of free iron, which is highly toxic, and iron storage to keep that toxicity going.[29]

NO. 6—HIGH-SENSITIVITY C-REACTIVE PROTEIN (HS-CRP)

The HS-CRP[30] is a test that measures a liver protein produced in response to inflammation in your body. It is a very sensitive marker for chronic inflammation, which is a hallmark of most chronic diseases. Ideally it should be below 1.0 mg/L, but the lower the better. I aim to keep mine around 0.2 mg/L. Anything over 3.0 mg/L is considered high risk for inflammatory diseases.

Conventional medicine will typically treat underlying inflammation with nonsteroidal anti-inflammatory drugs or corticosteroids. Patients with normal cholesterol but elevated CRP are also frequently prescribed a statin drug. None of these drug treatments address the underlying cause of the inflammation, and can do more harm than good in the long run.

Eating a healthy diet low in added sugars and higher in healthy fats, optimizing your vitamin D and omega-3, lowering your insulin level, and exercising on a regular basis will all help to address chronic inflammation. Certain herbs and supplements can also be useful, including astaxanthin, boswellia, bromelain, ginger, resveratrol, evening primrose, and curcumin.[31]

One drug option that is both safe and effective is low-dose naltrexone. Naltrexone is an opiate antagonist, originally developed for the treatment of opioid addiction. However, when taken at very low doses, it triggers endorphin production, which helps boost immune function, and has anti-inflammatory effects on the central nervous system.[32]

NO. 7—HOMOCYSTEINE

Homocysteine is an amino acid in your body and blood obtained primarily from meat consumption. Checking your homocysteine level is a great way to identify a vitamin B_6, B_9 (folate), or B_{12} deficiency.

Vitamins B_6, B_9, and B_{12} help convert homocysteine into methionine—a building block for proteins. If you don't get enough of these B vitamins, the conversion process is impaired and results in higher homocysteine. Conversely, when you increase intake of B_6, B_9, and B_{12}, your homocysteine level decreases.

Elevated homocysteine is a risk factor for heart disease, and when combined with a low omega-3 index, it's associated with an increased risk of brain atrophy and dementia.

Vitamins B_6, B_9, and B_{12} are also really important for cognition and mental health in general, so identifying and addressing a deficiency in these vitamins can go a long way toward warding off depression and other, even more serious, mental health conditions. If you do take folate and/or B$_{12}$ it would be best to take the methyl forms of these vitamins.

NO. 8—NMR LIPOPROFILE

One of the most important tests you can get to determine your heart disease risk is the NMR LipoProfile, which measures your low-density lipoprotein (LDL) particle number. This test also has other markers that can help determine if you have insulin resistance, which is a primary cause of elevated LDL particle number and increased heart disease risk.

Conventional doctors will usually only check your total cholesterol, LDL cholesterol, high-density lipoprotein (HDL) cholesterol, and triglycerides. However, these are not very accurate predictors for cardiovascular disease risk, as it's quite possible to have normal total cholesterol and/or normal LDL cholesterol yet have a high LDL particle number.

In a nutshell, it's not the amount of cholesterol that is the main risk factor for heart disease but rather it's the number of cholesterol-carrying LDL particles. The greater the number of LDL particles you have, the more likely it is that you also have oxidized LDL. Oxidized LDL is more harmful than normal nonoxidized LDL because it's smaller and denser. This allows it to penetrate the lining of your arteries, where it stimulates plaque formation.

Some groups, such as the National Lipid Association, have started to shift the focus toward LDL particle number instead of total and LDL cholesterol, but it still has not hit mainstream. Fortunately, if you know about it, you can take control of your health and either ask your doctor for this test or order it yourself.

There are several ways to test for your LDL particle number. The NMR LipoProfile is offered by a lab called LipoScience, and is the test used in most scientific studies on LDL particles. If your LDL particle number is high, chances are you have insulin and leptin resistance, as these are driving causes of high LDL particle numbers. Endotoxins in your gut will also increase your LDL particle number, and thyroid dysfunction may be at play as well.

2014 RULE GAVE PATIENTS DIRECT ACCESS TO LAB RESULTS

While there are hundreds of blood tests and other health screens available, the eight reviewed in this chapter are, I believe, among the most valuable, arming you with vital information you can then use to take proactive steps to protect and improve your health.

In case you've ever wondered if you can get your lab test results directly from the lab that conducted the testing, know that you do have that right. In 2014, the U.S. Department of Health and Human Services issued a final rule that grants patients (or a person they designate) direct access to their laboratory test reports without having to have them sent to a physician first.[33]

Clearly, doctors should not have exclusive rights to information about your body, but this wasn't always a guarantee. The final rule updated the Clinical Laboratory Improvement Amendments of 1988, allowing laboratories to give patients direct access to their lab results.

Even so, it's not always as simple as it should be to get your results without going through your doctor. Laboratories may require patients to make requests for lab results in writing, and they may charge you extra to mail or deliver them electronically.

Further, the rule states that most results must be made available to patients within 30 days of the completion of testing, so depending on the contentiousness of the lab, you may have to wait weeks to find out crucial health information. However, most tend to be fairly quick.

SUMMARY

- While studies suggest the health of Americans suffers due to excessive, unnecessary, and/or ineffective medical tests and treatments, certain lab tests can offer truly valuable clues about your health.

- Some of the most important tests are rarely ordered by conventional physicians. These include the omega-3 index, ferritin, RBC magnesium, homocysteine, LDL particle number, vitamin D, fasting insulin, and HS-CRP.

- You may also consider doing a GGT test. Not only will it tell you if you have liver damage, it's also an excellent marker for excess free iron and is a great indicator of your risk of sudden cardiac death.

- As of 2014, patients (or a person they designate) have the right to gain direct access to their laboratory test reports without having to have them sent to a physician first.

RESOURCES

Books

Fasting: An Exceptional Human Experience, by Randi Fredricks

The Circadian Code: Lose Weight, Supercharge Your Energy, and Sleep Well Every Night, by Dr. Satchin Panda

The Complete Guide to Fasting, by Dr. Jason Fung

The Diabetes Epidemic and You, by Dr. Joseph Kraft

Sauna Therapy for Detoxification and Healing, by Dr. Lawrence Wilson

Why We Sleep, by Dr. Matthew Walker

Films

Stink!
stinkmovie.com

Programs

The Walsh Detoxification Program
https://www.metabolicfitnesspro.com/walshdetox/

Products

Dr. Shade's Liver Sauce™, by Quicksilver Scientific (available only as part of the PushCatch™ Liver Detox package, at the time of this writing)
www.quicksilverscientific.com/pushcatch

Pure Power Organic Mitomix Seed Blend
https://products.mercola.com/mitomix-seed-blend/

Urban Moonshine bitters formulas
www.urbanmoonshine.com/

Blood tests

NMR LipoProfile, by LipoScience
www.truehealthlabs.com

Vitamin D and Omega-3 Index Test Kit, by GrassrootsHealth
daction.grassrootshealth.net/testing-options-vitamin-d/

Clinics

TrueNorth Health Center
www.healthpromoting.com

Apps and websites

Cronometer.com
www.cronometer.com/mercola

Environmental Working Group
www.EWG.org

MyCircadianClock
mycircadianclock.org

Vitamin D*calculator by GrassrootsHealth
grassrootshealth.net/?post_projects=dcalculator

ENDNOTES

Chapter 1

1. National Center for Chronic Disease Prevention and Health Promotion, "About Chronic Disease," Centers for Disease Control and Prevention, September 05, 2018, https://www.cdc.gov/chronicdisease/about/index.htm, accessed 10/19/18.

2. S. Hatfield, "Chronic Disease: Costly, Deadly, and Preventable," National Consumers League, http://www.nclnet.org/chronic_disease.

3. S. M. De La Monte, "Insulin Resistance and Alzheimer's Disease," *BMB Reports* 42, no. 8 (August 31, 2009): 475–81. https://www.ncbi.nlm.nih.gov /pubmed/19712582.

4. S. Gill and P. Satchidananda, "A Smartphone App Reveals Erratic Diurnal Eating Patterns in Humans that Can Be Modulated for Health Benefits," *Cell Metabolism* 22, no. 5 (2015): 789–98. DOI: 10.1016/j.cmet.2015.09.005.

5. T. Neltner and M. Maffini, "Generally Recognized as Secret: Chemicals Added to Food in the United States," NRDC Report, April 2014, https://www.nrdc.org /sites/default/files/safety-loophole-for-chemicals-in-food-report.pdf.

6. R. J. De Souza et al., "Intake of Saturated and Trans Unsaturated Fatty Acids and Risk of All Cause Mortality, Cardiovascular Disease, and Type 2 Diabetes: Systematic Review and Meta-analysis of Observational Studies," *BMJ*, August 11, 2015. DOI: 10.1136/bmj.h3978.

7. V. T. Samuel, K. F. Petersen, and G. J. Shulman, "Lipid-Induced Insulin Resistance: Unravelling the Mechanism," *Lancet* 375, no. 9733 (June 26, 2010): 2267–277. DOI: 10.1016/S0140-6736(10)60408-4.

8. K. Kavanagh et al., "Trans Fat Diet Induces Abdominal Obesity and Changes in Insulin Sensitivity in Monkeys," *Obesity* 15, no. 7 (July 2007): 1675–684. DOI: 10.1038/oby.2007.200.

9. M. C. Morris et al., "Dietary Fats and the Risk of Incident Alzheimer Disease," *Archives of Neurology* 60, no. 2 (February 2003): 194–200. https://www.ncbi .nlm.nih.gov/pubmed/12580703.

10. International Agency for Research on Cancer, "Evaluation of Five Organophophate Insecticides and Herbicides," IARC Monographs Volume 112, March 20, 2015, https://www.iarc.fr/en/media-centre/iarcnews/pdf/MonographVolume112.pdf, accessed 10/29/18.

11. M. Pall, "How to Approach the Challenge of Minimizing Non-Thermal Health Effects of Microwave Radiation from Electrical Devices," *International Journal of Innovative Research in Engineering and Management* 2, no. 5 (September 2015), https://www.researchgate.net/publication/283017154_How_to_Approach_the_Challenge_of_Minimizing_Non-Thermal_Health_Effects_of_Microwave_Radiation_from_Electrical_Devices, accessed 10/30/18.

12. M. Pall, "Electromagnetic Fields Act via Activation of Voltage-gated Calcium Channels to Produce Beneficial or Adverse Effects," *Journal of Cellular and Molecular Medicine* 17, no. 8 (2013): 958–65. DOI: 10.1111/jcmm.12088.

13. M. Pall, "Electromagnetic Fields Act Similarly in Plants as in Animals: Probable Activation of Calcium Channels via Their Voltage Sensor," *Current Chemical Biology* 10, no. 1 (2016): 74–82. DOI: 10.2174/2212796810666160419160433.

14. M. Pall, "Microwave Frequency Electromagnetic Fields (EMFs) Produce Widespread Neurophyschiatric Effects Including Depression," *Journal of Chemical Neuroanatomy* 75, part B (September 2016): 43–51. DOI: 10.1016/j.jchemneu.2015.08.001.

15. C. M. Benbrook, "Impacts of Genetically Engineered Crops on Pesticide Use in the U.S. — the First Sixteen Years," *Environmental Sciences Europe* 24, no. 1 (September 28, 2012): 24. DOI: 10.1186/2190-4715-24-24.

16. M. Pall, "Scientific Evidence Contradicts Findings and Assumptions of Canadian Safety Panel 6: Microwaves Act Through Voltage-Gated Calcium Channel Activation to Induce Biological Impacts at Non-Thermal Levels, Supporting a Paradigm Shift for Microwave/Lower Frequency Electromagnetic Field Action," *Reviews on Environmental Health* 30, no. 2 (2015): 99–116. DOI: 10.1515/reveh-2015-0001.

17. R. Sender, S. Fuchs, and R. Milo, "Revised Estimates for the Number of Human and Bacteria Cells in the Body." *PLoS One*, accessed 9/24/18. DOI: 10.1371/journal.pbio.1002533.

18. C. E. Forsythe et al., "Comparison of Low Fat and Low Carbohydrate Diets on Circulating Fatty Acid Composition and Markers of Inflammation," *Lipids* 43, no. 1 (2007): 65–77. DOI: 10.1007/s11745-007-3132-7.

19. Ibid.

20. N. Lane, *Power, Sex, Suicide: Mitochondria and the Meaning of Life* (Oxford: Oxford University Press, 2006).

21. S. Gill and P. Satchidananda, "A Smartphone App Reveals Erratic Diurnal Eating Patterns in Humans that Can Be Modulated for Health Benefits," *Cell Metabolism* 22, no. 5 (2015): 789–98. DOI: 10.1016/j.cmet.2015.09.005.

22. R. Pamploma, "Mitochondrial DNA Damage and Animal Longevity: Insights from Comparative Studies," *Journal of Aging and Research* 2011 (January 4, 2011). DOI: 10.4061/2011/807108.

Chapter 2

1. V. R. Young and N. S. Scrimshaw, "The Physiology of Starvation," *Scientific American* 225, no. 4 (October 1971): 14–21. https://www.ncbi.nlm.nih.gov /pubmed/5094959.

2. E. A. Genné-Bacon, "Thinking Evolutionarily about Obesity," *Yale Journal of Biology and Medicine* 87, no. 2 (June 6, 2014): 99–112, https://www.ncbi.nlm .nih.gov/pmc/articles/PMC4031802/.

3. R. Arbesmann, "Fasting and Prophecy in Pagan and Christian Antiquity," *Traditio* 7 (1951): 1–71. DOI: 10.1017/s0362152900015117.

4. J. D. M. Derrett and V. Macdermot, "The Cult of the Seer in the Ancient Middle East: A Contribution to Current Research on Hallucinations Drawn from Coptic and Other Texts," *Man* 8, no. 1 (1973): 146. https://www.jstor.org /stable/2800682. DOI: 10.2307/2800682.

5. M. M. Ali, *The Religion of Islam: A Comprehensive Discussion of the Sources, Principles and Practices of Islam* (Dublin, OH: Ahmadiyya Anjuman Ishaat Islam Lahore USA, 2014).

6. D. W. Mitchell and S. Jacoby, *Buddhism: Introducing the Buddhist Experience* (New York: Oxford University Press, 2014).

7. P. Dundas, *The Jains* (London: Routledge, 2010).

8. P. S. Jaini, *Collected Papers on Buddhist Studies* (Delhi: Motilal Banarsidass Publishers, 2001).

9. L. Kohn, *Daoist Body Cultivation: Traditional Models and Contemporary Practices* (Magdalena, N.M.: Three Pine Press, 2006).

10. S. Arthur, *Early Daoist Dietary Practices - Examining Ways to Health and Longevity* (Lanham, MD: Lexington Books, 2015).

11. S. Arthur, "Eating Your Way to Immortality: Early Daoist Self-Cultivation Diets," *Journal of Daoist Studies* 2, no. 1 (2009): 32–63. DOI: 10.1353/dao.2009.0001.

12. T. Keneally, *Three Famines: Starvation and Politics* (New York: PublicAffairs, 2011).

13. S. A. Russell, *Hunger: An Unnatural History* (New York: Basic Books, 2008).

14. J. L. Brockington, *The Sanskrit Epics* (Leiden, The Netherlands: Brill, 1998).

15. P. O'Malley, *Biting at the Grave: The Irish Hunger Strikes and the Politics of Despair* (Boston: Beacon Press, 2001).

16. S. Ramachandran, "India's Forgotten Fast," I Manipur, http://imanipur .blogspot.com/2011/09/indias-forgotten-fast.html.

17. N. G. Wilson, Ed., *Encyclopedia of Ancient Greece* (London: Psychology Press, 2006).

18. L. B. Hazzard, *Scientific Fasting: The Ancient and Modern Key to Health* (Whitefish, MT: Kessinger Publishing, 1996).

19. S. Graham, *The Greatest Health Discovery: Natural Hygiene and Its Evolution, Past, Present & Future* (Chicago: Natural Hygiene Press, 1972).

20. H. M. Shelton, *Fasting Can Save Your Life*. 2nd ed. (Chicago: Natural Hygiene Press, 1981).

Chapter 3

1. S. Furmli et al., "Therapeutic Use of Intermittent Fasting for People with Type 2 Diabetes as an Alternative to Insulin," *BMJ Case Reports* 2018. DOI: 10.1136/bcr-2017-221854.

2. Joseph Mercola, "Autophagy Finally Considered for Disease Treatment," https://articles.mercola.com/sites/articles/archive/2018/06/27/autophagy-health-benefits.aspx.

3. National Institutes of Health, "4. The Adult Stem Cell," https://stemcells.nih.gov/info/2001report/chapter4. htm.http://stemcells.nih.gov/info/basics/pages/basics4.aspx.

4. C. W. Cheng et al., "Prolonged Fasting Reduces IGF-1/PKA to Promote Hematopoietic-Stem-Cell-Based Regeneration and Reverse Immunosuppression," *Cell Stem Cell* 14, no. 6 (June 5, 2014): 810–23. https://www.sciencedirect.com/science/article/pii/S1934590914001519.

5. M. M. Mihaylova et al., "Fasting Activates Fatty Acid Oxidation to Enhance Intestinal Stem Cell Function during Homeostasis and Aging," *Cell Stem Cell* 22, no. 5 (May 3, 2018): 769–78. DOI: 10.1016/j.stem.2018.04.001.

6. R. Morello-Frosch et al., "Environmental Chemicals in an Urban Population of Pregnant Women and Their Newborns from San Francisco," *Environmental Science and Technology* 50, no. 22 (2016): 12464–12472. DOI: 10.1021/acs.est.6b03492.

7. Environmental Working Group, "Body Burden: The Pollution in Newborns," July 14, 2005, https://www.ewg.org/research/body-burden-pollution-newborns, accessed 10/29/18.

8. D. L. Frape et al., "Diurnal Trends in Responses of Blood Plasma Concentrations of Glucose, Insulin, and C-peptide following High- and Low-fat Meals and Their Relation to Fat Metabolism in Healthy Middle-aged Volunteers," *British Journal of Nutrition* 77, no. 4 (April 1997): 523–35. https://www.ncbi.nlm.nih.gov/pubmed/9155503; M. Gibbs et al., "Diurnal Postprandial Responses to Low and High Glycaemic Index Mixed Meals," *Clinical Nutrition* 33, no. 5 (October 2014): 889–94. DOI: 10.1016/j.clnu.2013.09.018; C. R. Marinac et al., "Frequency and Circadian Timing of Eating May Influence Biomarkers of Inflammation and Insulin Resistance Associated with Breast Cancer Risk," *PLoS One* 10, no. 8 (August 25, 2015). DOI: 10.1371/journal.pone.0136240; L. Morgan et al., "Circadian Aspects of Postprandial Metabolism," *Chronobiology International* 20, no. 5 (2003): 795–808. DOI: 10.1081/cbi-120024218; K. S. Polonsky, B. D. Given, and E. Van Cauter, "Twenty-four-hour Profiles and Pulsatile Patterns of Insulin Secretion in Normal and Obese Subjects," *Journal of Clinical Investigation* 81, no. 2 (1988): 442–48. DOI: 10.1172/jci113339.

9. Joseph Mercola, "Gut Microbiome May Be a Game-Changer for Cancer Prevention and Treatment," https://articles.mercola.com/sites/articles/archive/2018/06/11/gut-microbiome-game-changer.aspx.

10. R. Shen et al., "Neuronal Energy-sensing Pathway Promotes Energy Balance by Modulating Disease Tolerance," *Proceedings of the National Academy of Sciences* 113, no. 23 (2016). DOI: 10.1073/pnas.1606106113.

11. J. Fung and J. Moore, *The Complete Guide to Fasting: Heal Your Body Through Intermittent, Alternate-Day, and Extended Fasting* (Las Vegas: Victory Belt Publishing, 2016).

12. J. Volek and S. D. Phinney, *The Art and Science of Low Carbohydrate Living: An Expert Guide to Making the Life-saving Benefits of Carbohydrate Restriction Sustainable and Enjoyable* (Lexington, KY: Beyond Obesity, 2011).

13. D. Y. Kim et al., "Ketone Bodies Are Protective against Oxidative Stress in Neocortical Neurons," *Journal of Neurochemistry* 101, no. 5 (June 2007): 1316–326. DOI: 10.1111/j.1471-4159.2007.04483.x.

14. D. Stipp, "Is Fasting Good for You?" *Scientific American* 24 (March 5, 2015): 56–57. DOI: 10.1038/scientificamericansecrets0315-56.

15. M. A. McNally and A. L. Hartman, "Ketone Bodies in Epilepsy," *Journal of Neurochemistry* 121, no. 1 (February 7, 2012): 28–35. DOI: 10.1111/j.1471 -4159.2012.07670.x.

16. J. Moore and E. C. Westman, *Keto Clarity* (Las Vegas: Victory Belt Publishing, 2014).

17. A. J. Brown, "Low-Carb Diets, Fasting and Euphoria: Is There a Link between Ketosis and γ-hydroxybutyrate (GHB)?" *Medical Hypotheses* 68, no. 2 (2007): 268–71. DOI: 10.1016/j.mehy.2006.07.043.

18. S. Bair, "Intermittent Fasting: Try This at Home for Brain Health," Stanford Law School, https://law.stanford.edu/2015/01/09/lawandbiosciences-2015-01-09 -intermittent-fasting-try-this-at-home-for-brain-health/, accessed 9/23/18; B. Martin, M. P. Mattson, and S. Maudsley, "Caloric Restriction and Intermittent Fasting: Two Potential Diets for Successful Brain Aging," *Ageing Research Reviews* 5, no. 3 (2006): 332–53. DOI: 10.1016/j.arr.2006.04.002.

19. S. Komanduri et al., "Prevalence and Risk Factors of Heart Failure in the USA: NHANES 2013 – 2014 Epidemiological Follow-up Study," *Journal of Community Hospital Internal Medicine Perspectives* 7, no. 1 (January 2017): 15–20. DOI: 10.1080/20009666.2016.1264696.

20. E. Renguet et al., "Erratum: The Regulation of Insulin-Stimulated Cardiac Glucose Transport via Protein Acetylation," *Frontiers in Cardiovascular Medicine* 5 (June 12, 2018). DOI: 10.3389/fcvm.2018.00103.

21. Q. G. Karwi et al., "Loss of Metabolic Flexibility in the Failing Heart," *Frontiers in Cardiovascular Medicine* 5 (2018). DOI: 10.3389/fcvm.2018.00068.

22. R. J. Bing et al., "Metabolism of the Human Heart: II. Studies on Fat, Ketone and Amino Acid Metabolism," *American Journal of Medicine* 16, no. 4 (April 1954): 504–15. https://www.sciencedirect.com/science/article /pii/0002934354903654. DOI: 10.1016/0002-9343(54)90365-4.

23. P. Puchalska and P. Crawford, "Multi-dimensional Roles of Ketone Bodies in Fuel Metabolism, Signaling, and Therapeutics," *Cell Metabolism* 25, no. 2 (February 7, 2017): 262–84. DOI: 10.1016/j.cmet.2016.12.022.

Chapter 4

1. R. C. Shoemaker, *Surviving Mold: Life in the Era of Dangerous Buildings* (Baltimore: Otter Bay Books, 2010).

2 R. A. Lordo, K. T. Dinh, and J. G. Schwemberger, "Semivolatile Organic Compounds in Adipose Tissue: Estimated Averages for the US Population and Selected Subpopulations," *American Journal of Public Health* 86, no. 9 (1996): 1253–259. DOI: 10.2105/ajph.86.9.1253.

3. J. E. Orban et al., "Dioxins and Dibenzofurans in Adipose Tissue of the General US Population and Selected Subpopulations," *American Journal of Public Health* 84, no. 3 (1994): 439–45. DOI: 10.2105/ajph.84.3.439.

4. D. Main, "Glyphosate Now the Most-Used Agricultural Chemical Ever," *Newsweek* May 19, 2016, https://www.newsweek.com/glyphosate-now-most -used-agricultural-chemical-ever-422419.

5. K. A. Varady et al., "Alternate Day Fasting for Weight Loss in Normal Weight and Overweight Subjects: A Randomized Controlled Trial," *Nutrition Journal* 12, no. 1 (2013). DOI: 10.1186/1475-2891-12-146.

6. I. Ahmet et al., "Chronic Alternate-Day Fasting Results in Reduced Diastolic Compliance and Diminished Systolic Reserve in Rats," *Journal of Cardiac Failure* 16, no. 10 (October 2016): 843–53. https://www.ncbi.nlm.nih.gov /pubmed/20932467.

Chapter 5

1. A. M. Elsakka et al., "Management of Glioblastoma Multiforme in a Patient Treated with Ketogenic Metabolic Therapy and Modified Standard of Care: A 24-Month Follow-Up," *Frontiers in Nutrition* 5, no. 20 (March 29, 2018). DOI: 10.3389/fnut.2018.00020.

Chapter 6

1. K. Breivik et al., "Primary Sources of Selected POPs: Regional and Global Scale Emission Inventories," *Environmental Pollution* 128, no. 1–2 (2004): 3–16. DOI: 10.1016/j.envpol.2003.08.031.

2. A. Sjödin et al., "Polybrominated Diphenyl Ethers, Polychlorinated Biphenyls, and Persistent Pesticides in Serum from the National Health and Nutrition Examination Survey: 2003–2008," *Environmental Science & Technology* 48, no. 1 (2013): 753–60. DOI: 10.1021/es4037836.

3. D. G. Patterson Jr. et al., "Levels in the U.S. Population of Those Persistent Organic Pollutants (2003–2004) Included in the Stockholm Convention or in Other Long-Range Transboundary Air Pollution Agreements," *Environmental Science & Technology* 43, no. 4 (2009): 1211–218. DOI: 10.1021/es801966w.

4. P. J. Landrigan, "Pesticides and Polychlorinated Biphenyls (PCBs): An Analysis of the Evidence that They Impair Children's Neurobehavioral Development," *Molecular Genetics and Metabolism* 73, no. 1 (2001): 11–17. DOI: 10.1006 /mgme.2001.3177.

5. E. Jackson et al., "Adipose Tissue as a Site of Toxin Accumulation," *Comprehensive Physiology* 7, no. 4 (2017): 1085–135. DOI: 10.1002/cphy.c160038.

6. D. G. Patterson Jr. et al., "Levels in the U.S. Population of Those Persistent Organic Pollutants (2003–2004) Included in the Stockholm Convention or in Other Long-Range Transboundary Air Pollution Agreements," 1211–218.

7. Y. Y. Qin et al., "Persistent Organic Pollutants and Heavy Metals in Adipose Tissues of Patients with Uterine Leiomyomas and the Association of These Pollutants with Seafood Diet, BMI, and Age," *Environmental Science and Pollution Research* 17, no. 1 (October 27, 2009): 229–240. https://link.springer .com/article/10.1007/s11356-009-0251-0, accessed 10/19/18.

8. V. Bornemann et al., "Intestinal Metabolism and Bioaccumulation of Sucralose in Adipose Tissue in the Rat," *Journal of Toxicology and Environmental Health, Part A* 81, no. 18 (2018): 913–923. DOI: 10.1080/15287394.2018.1502560.

9. M. Haranczyk et al., "On Enumeration of Congeners of Common Persistent Organic Pollutants," *Environmental Pollution* 158, no. 8 (2010): 2786–789. DOI: 10.1016/j.envpol.2010.05.011.

10. Environmental Protection Agency, "Persistant Organic Pollutants: A Global Issue, A Global Response," 2002, updated in December, 2009. https://www .epa.gov/international-cooperation/persistent-organic-pollutants-global-issue -global-response, accessed December 6, 2018.

11. D. H. Lee et al., "A Strong Dose-Response Relation between Serum Concentrations of Persistent Organic Pollutants and Diabetes: Results from the National Health and Examination Survey 1999–2002," *Diabetes Care* 29, no. 7 (July 2006): 1638–644. DOI: 10.2337/dc06-0543.

12. M. C. Petriello, B. Newsome, and B. Hennig, "Influence of Nutrition in PCB-Induced Vascular Inflammation," *Environmental Science and Pollution Research* 21, no. 10 (2013): 6410–418. DOI: 10.1007/s11356-013-1549-5.

13. J. Kumar et al., "Persistent Organic Pollutants and Inflammatory Markers in a Cross-Sectional Study of Elderly Swedish People: The PIVUS Cohort," *Environmental Health Perspectives* 122, no. 9 (2014): 977–83. DOI: 10.1289 /ehp.1307613.

14. D. Costantini et al., "Oxidative Stress in Relation to Reproduction, Contaminants, Gender and Age in a Long-Lived Seabird," *Oecologia* 175, no. 4 (2014): 1107–116. DOI: 10.1007/s00442-014-2975-x.

15. M. A. Hyman, "Environmental Toxins, Obesity, and Diabetes: An Emerging Risk Factor," *Alternative Therapies in Health and Medicine* 16, no. 2 (March/ April 2010): 56–8. https://www.ncbi.nlm.nih.gov/pubmed/20232619.

16. S. E. Kahn, R. L. Hull, and K. M. Utzschneider, "Mechanisms Linking Obesity to Insulin Resistance and Type 2 Diabetes," *Nature* 444, no. 7121 (2006): 840–46. DOI: 10.1038/nature05482.

17. D. H. Lee et al., "Low Dose Organochlorine Pesticides and Polychlorinated Biphenyls Predict Obesity, Dyslipidemia, and Insulin Resistance among People Free of Diabetes," *PLoS One* 6, no. 1 (2011). DOI: 10.1371/journal .pone.0015977.

18. C. C. Kuo et al., "Environmental Chemicals and Type 2 Diabetes: An Updated Systematic Review of the Epidemiologic Evidence," *Current Diabetes Reports* 13, no. 6 (2013): 831–49. DOI: 10.1007/s11892-013-0432-6.

19. R. Rezg et al., "Bisphenol A and Human Chronic Diseases: Current Evidences, Possible Mechanisms, and Future Perspectives," *Environment International* 64 (2014): 83–90. DOI: 10.1016/j.envint.2013.12.007.

20. H. K. Lee and Y. K. Pak, "Persistent Organic Pollutants, Mitochondrial Dysfunction, and Metabolic Syndrome," *Mitochondrial Dysfunction Caused by Drugs and Environmental Toxicants* (2018): 691–707. DOI: 10.1002/9781119329725.ch44.

21. K. Fry and M. C. Power, "Persistent Organic Pollutants and Mortality in the United States, NHANES 1999–2011," *Environmental Health* 16, no. 1 (2017). DOI: 10.1186/s12940-017-0313-6.

22. S. H. Safe, "Polychlorinated Biphenyls (PCBs): Environmental Impact, Biochemical and Toxic Responses, and Implications for Risk Assessment," *Critical Reviews in Toxicology* 24, no. 2 (1994): 87–149. DOI: 10.3109/10408449409049308.

23. Centers for Disease Control and Prevention, "Toxic Substances Portal - Polybrominated Diphenyl Ethers (PBDEs)," January 21, 2015, https://www.atsdr.cdc.gov/phs/phs.asp?id=1449&tid=183, accessed 10/20/18.

24. M. Frederiksen et al., "Human Internal and External Exposure to PBDEs – A Review of Levels and Sources," *International Journal of Hygiene and Environmental Health* 212, no. 2 (2009): 109–34. DOI: 10.1016/j.ijheh.2008.04.005.

25. C. Chevrier et al. "Childhood Exposure to Polybrominated Diphenyl Ethers and Neurodevelopment at Six Years of Age," *NeuroToxicology* 54 (2016): 81–88. DOI: 10.1016/j.neuro.2016.03.002.

26. G. Ding et al., "Association between Prenatal Exposure to Polybrominated Diphenyl Ethers and Young Children's Neurodevelopment in China," *Environmental Research* 142 (2015): 104–11. DOI: 10.1016/j.envres.2015.06.008.

27. M. P. Vélez, T. E. Arbuckle, and W. D. Fraser, "Maternal Exposure to Perfluorinated Chemicals and Reduced Fecundity: The MIREC Study," *Human Reproduction* 30, no. 3 (2015): 701–09. DOI: 10.1093/humrep/deu350.

28. Environmental Protection Agency, "Learn about Polychlorinated Biphenyls (PCBs)," April 13, 2018, https://www.epa.gov/pcbs/learn-about-polychlorinated-biphenyls-pcbs.

29. United Nations Environment Programme, "Stockholm Convention on Persistent Organic Pollutants (POPs) as Amended in 2009," 2009.

30. M. Cave et al., "Polychlorinated Biphenyls, Lead, and Mercury Are Associated with Liver Disease in American Adults: NHANES 2003–2004," *Environmental Health Perspectives* 118, no. 12 (2010): 1735–742. DOI: 10.1289/ehp.1002720.

31. P. A. Eubig et al., "Lead and PCBs as Risk Factors for Attention Deficit/ Hyperactivity Disorder," *Environmental Health Perspectives* 118, no. 12 (2010): 1654–667. DOI: 10.1289/ehp.0901852.

32. S. A. Kim et al., "Associations of Organochlorine Pesticides and Polychlorinated Biphenyls with Total, Cardiovascular, and Cancer Mortality in Elders with Differing Fat Mass," *Environmental Research*. 138 (2015): 1–7. DOI: 10.1016/j .envres.2015.01.021.

33. Y. S. Lin et al., "Environmental Exposure to Dioxin-Like Compounds and the Mortality Risk in the U.S. Population," *International Journal of Hygiene and Environmental Health* 215, no. 6 (2012): 541–546. DOI: 10.1016/j .ijheh.2012.02.006.

34. K. Fry and M. C. Power, "Persistent Organic Pollutants and Mortality in the United States, NHANES 1999–2011," *Environmental Health* 16, no. 1 (2017):105. DOI:10.1186/s12940-017-0313-6.

35. R. S. Pardini, "Polychlorinated Biphenyls (PCB): Effect on Mitochondrial Enzyme Systems," *Bulletin of Environmental Contamination and Toxicology* 6, no. 6 (1971): 539–45. DOI: 10.1007/bf01796863.

36. M. C. Petriello et al., "Modulation of Persistent Organic Pollutant Toxicity through Nutritional Intervention: Emerging Opportunities in Biomedicine and Environmental Remediation," *Science of the Total Environment* 491–492 (2014): 11–16. DOI: 10.1016/j.scitotenv.2014.01.109.

37. M. C. Petriello, B. Newsome, and B. Hennig, "Influence of Nutrition in PCB-Induced Vascular Inflammation," *Environmental Science and Pollution Research* 21, no. 10 (2013): 6410–418. DOI: 10.1007/s11356-013-1549-5.

38. O. Krupkova, J. Handa, M. Hlavna, et al., "The Natural Polyphenol Epigallocatechin Gallate Protects Intervertebral Disc Cells from Oxidative Stress," *Oxidative Medicine and Cellular Longevity* 2016 (2016): 7031397. DOI: 10.1155/2016/7031397.

39. Centers for Disease Control and Prevention, "Arsenic Toxicity: Where Is Arsenic Found?," https://www.atsdr.cdc.gov/csem/csem.asp?csem=1&po=5, accessed 10/20/18.

40. Centers for Disease Control and Prevention, "Toxic Substances Portal – Copper," January 21, 2015, https://www.atsdr.cdc.gov/phs/phs .asp?id=204&tid=37, accessed 10/20/18.

41. R. Chowdhury et al., "Environmental Toxic Metal Contaminants and Risk of Cardiovascular Disease: Systematic Review and Meta-analysis," *BMJ* 2018. DOI: 10.1136/bmj.k3310.

42. National Center for Complementary and Integrative Health, "Questions and Answers: The NIH Trials of EDTA Chelation Therapy for Coronary Heart Disease," October 11, 2016, https://nccih.nih.gov/health/chelation/TACT -questions; https://www.newsmax.com/Health/dr-crandall/chelation-heart -attack-diabetes-angioplasty/2018/02/09/id/842527/, accessed 10/20/18.

43. R. Walford, "Physiologic Changes in Humans Subjected to Severe, Selective Calorie Restriction for Two Years in Biosphere 2: Health, Aging, and Toxicological Perspectives," *Toxicological Sciences* 52, no. 2 (1999): 61–65. DOI: 10.1093/toxsci/52.2.61.

44. W. E. Dale, T. B. Gaines, and W. J. Hayes, "Storage and Excretion of DDT in Starved Rats." *Toxicology and Applied Pharmacology* 4, no. 1 (1962): 89–106. DOI: 10.1016/0041-008x(62)90078-9.

45. G. M. Findlay and A. S. W. Defreitas, "DDT Movement from Adipocyte to Muscle Cell during Lipid Utilization." *Nature* 229, no. 5279 (1971): 63–65. DOI: 10.1038/229063a0.

46. D. C. Villeneuve, "The Effect of Food Restriction on the Redistribution of Hexachlorobenzene in the Rat," *Toxicology and Applied Pharmacology* 31, no. 2 (1975): 313–19. DOI: 10.1016/0041-008x(75)90167-2.

47. O. Hue et al., "Increased Plasma Levels of Toxic Pollutants Accompanying Weight Loss Induced by Hypocaloric Diet or by Bariatric Surgery," *Obesity Surgery* 16, no. 9 (2006): 1145–154. DOI: 10.1381/096089206778392356.

48. M. J. Kim et al., "Fate and Complex Pathogenic Effects of Dioxins and Polychlorinated Biphenyls in Obese Subjects Before and After Drastic Weight Loss," *Environmental Health Perspectives* 119, no. 3 (2011): 377–83. DOI: 10.1289/ehp.1002848.

49. M. Rosenbaum and R. L. Leibel, "Adaptive Thermogenesis in Humans," *International Journal of Obesity* 34, no. 1 (October 2010): 47–55. DOI: 10.1038/ijo.2010.184.

50. A. Tremblay et al., "Thermogenesis and Weight Loss in Obese Individuals: A Primary Association with Organochlorine Pollution," *International Journal of Obesity* 28, no. 7 (2004): 936–39. DOI: 10.1038/sj.ijo.0802527.

51. C. Pelletier, P. Imbeault, and A. Tremblay, "Energy Balance and Pollution by Organochlorines and Polychlorinated Biphenyls," *Obesity Reviews* 4, no. 1 (2003): 17–24. DOI: 10.1046/j.1467-789x.2003.00085.x.

52. J. Chevrier et al., "Body Weight Loss Increases Plasma and Adipose Tissue Concentrations of Potentially Toxic Pollutants in Obese Individuals," *International Journal of Obesity* 24, no. 10 (2000): 1272–278. DOI: 10.1038/sj.ijo.0801380.

53. C. Charlier, C. I. Desaive, and G. Plomteux, "Human Exposure to Endocrine Disrupters: Consequences of Gastroplasty on Plasma Concentration of Toxic Pollutants," *International Journal of Obesity* 26, no. 11 (2002): 1465–468. DOI: 10.1038/sj.ijo.0802144.

54. C. Pelletier et al., "Associations between Weight Loss-Induced Changes in Plasma Organochlorine Concentrations, Serum T3 Concentration, and Resting Metabolic Rate," *Toxicological Sciences* 67, no. 1 (2002): 46–51. DOI: 10.1093/toxsci/67.1.46.

55. P. Imbeault et al., "Weight Loss-induced Rise in Plasma Pollutant Is Associated with Reduced Skeletal Muscle Oxidative Capacity," *American Journal of Physiology-Endocrinology and Metabolism* 282, no. 3 (2002). DOI: 10.1152/ajpendo.00394.2001.

56. V. Mildaziene, "Multiple Effects of 2,2`,5,5`-Tetrachlorobiphenyl on Oxidative Phosphorylation in Rat Liver Mitochondria," *Toxicological Sciences* 65, no. 2 (2002): 220–27. DOI: 10.1093/toxsci/65.2.220.

57. R. L. Leibel, M. Rosenbaum, and J. Hirsch, "Changes in Energy Expenditure Resulting from Altered Body Weight," *New England Journal of Medicine* 332, no. 10 (March 9, 1995): 621–28. DOI: 10.1056/NEJM199503093321001.

58. E. Doucet et al., "Evidence for the Existence of Adaptive Thermogenesis During Weight Loss," *British Journal of Nutrition* 85, no. 06 (2001): 715. DOI: 10.1079 /bjn2001348.

59. Y. Ohmiya and K. Nakai, "Effect of Starvation on Excretion, Distribution and Metabolism of DDT in Mice," *Tohoku Journal of Experimental Medicine* 122, no. 2 (1977): 143–53. DOI: 10.1620/tjem.122.143.

60. A. Aguilar, A. Borrell, and T. Pastor, "Biological Factors Affecting Variability of Persistent Pollutant Levels in Cetaceans," *Journal of Cetacean Research and Management* (January 1999): 83–116. https://www.researchgate .net/publication/235334517_Biological_factors_affecting_variability_of _persistent_pollutant_levels_in_cetaceans.

61. C. Lydersen et al., "Blood Is a Poor Substrate for Monitoring Pollution Burdens in Phocid Seals," *Science of The Total Environment* 292, no. 3 (2002): 193–203. DOI: 10.1016/s0048-9697(01)01121-4.

62. C. Debier et al., "Dynamics of PCB Transfer from Mother to Pup during Lactation in UK Grey Seals Halichoerus Grypus: Differences in PCB Profile between Compartments of Transfer and Changes during the Lactation Period," *Marine Ecology Progress Series* 247 (2003): 249–56. DOI: 10.3354 /meps247249.

63. C. Lydersen et al., "Blood Is a Poor Substrate for Monitoring Pollution Burdens in Phocid Seals," *Science of The Total Environment* 292, no. 3 (2002): 193–203. DOI: 10.1016/s0048-9697(01)01121-4.

64. C. Debier et al., "Mobilization of PCBs from Blubber to Blood in Northern Elephant Seals (Mirounga Angustirostris) during the Post-Weaning Fast," *Aquatic Toxicology* 80, no. 2 (2006): 149–57. DOI: 10.1016/j .aquatox.2006.08.002.

65. M. G. Peterson et al., "Serum POP Concentrations Are Highly Predictive of Inner Blubber Concentrations at Two Extremes of Body Condition in Northern Elephant Seals," *Environmental Pollution* 218 (2016): 651–63. DOI: 10.1016/j.envpol.2016.07.052.

66. J. Chevrier et al., "Body Weight Loss Increases Plasma and Adipose Tissue Concentrations of Potentially Toxic Pollutants in Obese Individuals," *International Journal of Obesity* 24, no. 10 (2000): 1272–278. DOI: 10.1038 /sj.ijo.0801380.

67. P. Imbeault et al., "Weight Loss-induced Rise in Plasma Pollutant Is Associated with Reduced Skeletal Muscle Oxidative Capacity," *American Journal of Physiology-Endocrinology and Metabolism* 282, no. 3 (2002). DOI: 10.1152 /ajpendo.00394.2001.

68. R. J. Jandacek et al., "Effects of Yo-Yo Diet, Caloric Restriction, and Olestra on Tissue Distribution of Hexachlorobenzene," *American Journal of Physiology-Gastrointestinal and Liver Physiology* 288, no. 2 (2005). DOI: 10.1152 /ajpgi.00285.2004.

69. M. L. Kortelainin, "Hyperthermia Deaths in Finland in 1970–1986," *American Journal of Forensic Medicine and Pathology* 12, no. 2 (June, 1991): 115–8. DOI: 10.1097/00000433-199106000-00006.

70. A. Kenttämies and K. Karkola, "Death in Sauna," *Journal of Forensic Science* 53 (2008): 724–729. DOI: 10.1111/j.1556-4029.2008.00703.x.

Chapter 7

1. K. Gabel et al., "Effects of 8-hour Time Restricted Feeding on Body Weight and Metabolic Disease Risk Factors in Obese Adults: A Pilot Study," *Nutrition and Healthy Aging* 4, no. 4 (2018): 345–53. DOI: 10.3233/nha-170036.

2. P. Puchalska and P. A. Crawford, "Multi-dimensional Roles of Ketone Bodies in Fuel Metabolism, Signaling, and Therapeutics," *Cell Metabolism* 25, no. 2 (2017): 262–84. DOI: 10.1016/j.cmet.2016.12.022.

3. J. S. Volek, T. Noakes, and S. D. Phinney, "Rethinking Fat as a Fuel for Endurance Exercise," *European Journal of Sport Science* 15, no. 1 (2014): 13–20. DOI: 10.1080/17461391.2014.959564.

4. K. A. Varady and M. K. Hellerstein, "Do Calorie Restriction or Alternate-Day Fasting Regimens Modulate Adipose Tissue Physiology in a Way that Reduces Chronic Disease Risk?" *Nutrition Reviews* 66, no. 6 (June 2008): 333–42. DOI: 10.1111/j.1753-4887.2008.00041.x.

5. G. F. Cahill, "Fuel Metabolism in Starvation," *Annual Review of Nutrition* 26, no. 1 (2006): 1–22. DOI: 10.1146/annurev.nutr.26.061505.111258.

6. L. B. Gano, M. Patel, and J. M. Rho, "Ketogenic Diets, Mitochondria, and Neurological Diseases," *Journal of Lipid Research* 55, no. 11 (2014): 2211–228. DOI: 10.1194/jlr.r048975.

7. Y. Kashiwya, M. T. King, and R. L. Veech, "Substrate Signaling by Insulin: A Ketone Bodies Ratio Mimics Insulin Action in Heart," *American Journal of Cardiology* 80, no. 3A (August 4, 1997): 50A–64A. https://www.ncbi.nlm.nih .gov/pubmed/9293956.

8. H. A. Krebs and R. L. Veech, "Pyridine Nucleotide Interrelations. In: The Energy Level and Metabolic Control in Mitochondria," *Adriatica Editrice* 1969, 329–84.

9. W. Curtis et al., "Mitigation of Damage from Reactive Oxygen Species and Ionizing Radiation by Ketone Body Esters," *Oxford Medicine Online* 2016. DOI: 10.1093/med/9780190497996.003.0027.

10. Y. Yang and A. A. Sauve, "NAD(+) Metabolism: Bioenergetics, Signaling and Manipulation for Therapy," *Biochimica Et Biophysica Acta* 1864, no. 12 (December 2016): 1787–800. DOI: 10.1016/j.bbapap.2016.06.014.

11. W. Ying, "NAD+/NADH and NADP+/NADPH in Cellular Functions and Cell Death: Regulation and Biological Consequences," *Antioxidants & Redox Signaling* 10, no. 2 (2008): 179–206. DOI: 10.1089/ars.2007.1672.

12. J. P. Fessel and W. M. Oldham, "Pyridine Dinucleotides from Molecules to Man," *Antioxidants & Redox Signaling* 28, no. 3 (2018): 180–212. DOI: 10.1089/ars.2017.7120.

13. M. N. Harvie et al., "The Effect of Intermittent Energy and Carbohydrate Restriction v. Daily Energy Restriction on Weight Loss and Metabolic Disease Risk Markers in Overweight Women," *British Journal of Nutrition* 110, no. 8 (October 2013): 1534–547. DOI: 10.1017/S0007114513000792.

14. H. Arquin et al., "Short- and Long-Term Effects of Continuous versus Intermittent Restrictive Diet Approaches on Body Composition and the Metabolic Profile in Overweight and Obese Postmenopausal Women: A Pilot Study," *Menopause New York* 19, no. 8 (August 2012): 870–76. DOI: 10.1097/gme.0b013e318250a287.

15. N. Halberg et al., "Effect of Intermittent Fasting and Refeeding on Insulin Action in Healthy Men," *Journal of Applied Physiology* 99, no. 6 (2005): 2128–136. DOI: 10.1152/japplphysiol.00683.2005.

16. M. N. Harvie et al., "The Effects of Intermittent or Continuous Energy Restriction on Weight Loss and Metabolic Disease Risk Markers: A Randomized Trial in Young Overweight Women," *International Journal of Obesity* 35, no. 5 (May 2011): 714–27. DOI: 10.1038/ijo.2010.171.

17. V. Ziaee et al., "The Changes of Metabolic Profile and Weight During Ramadan Fasting," *Singapore Medical Journal* 47, no. 5 (May 2006): 409–14. https://www.ncbi.nlm.nih.gov/pubmed/16645692.

18. M. A. Faris et al., "Intermittent Fasting during Ramadan Attenuates Proinflammatory Cytokines and Immune Cells in Healthy Subjects," *Nutritional Research* 32, no. 12 (December 2012): 947–55. DOI: 10.1016/j.nutres.2012.06.021.

19. J. B. Johnson et al., "Alternate Day Calorie Restriction Improves Clinical Findings and Reduces Markers of Oxidative Stress and Inflammation in Overweight Adults with Moderate Asthma," *Free Radical Biology & Medicine* 42, no. 5 (March 2007): 665–74. DOI: 10.1016/j.freeradbiomed.2006.12.005.

20. K. K. Hoddy et al., "Meal Timing during Alternate Day Fasting: Impact on Body Weight and Cardiovascular Disease Risk in Obese Adults," *Obesity* 22, no. 12 (December 2014): 2524–531. DOI: 10.1002/oby.20909.

21. M. C. Klempel et al., "Intermittent Fasting Combined with Calorie Restriction Is Effective for Weight Loss and Cardio-Protection in Obese Women," *Nutrition Journal* 11, no. 1 (2012). DOI: 10.1186/1475-2891-11-98.

22. B. D. Horne et al., "Relation of Routine, Periodic Fasting to Risk of Diabetes Mellitus, and Coronary Artery Disease in Patients Undergoing Coronary Angiography," *American Journal of Cardiology* 109, no. 11 (June 1, 2012): 1558–562. DOI: 10.1016/j.amjcard.2012.01.379.

23. M. Boutant et al., "SIRT1 Gain of Function Does Not Mimic or Enhance the Adaptations to Intermittent Fasting," *Cell Reports* 14, no. 9 (March 8, 2016): 2068–075. DOI: 10.1016/j.celrep.2016.02.007.

24. K. A. Varady et al., "Alternate Day Fasting for Weight Loss in Normal Weight and Overweight Subjects: A Randomized Controlled Trial," *Nutrition Journal* 12, no. 1 (2013). DOI: 10.1186/1475-2891-12-146.

25. M. P. Wegman et al., "Practicality of Intermittent Fasting in Humans and Its Effect on Oxidative Stress and Genes Related to Aging and Metabolism," *Rejuvenation Research* 18, no. 2 (April 1, 2015): 162–72. DOI: 10.1089/rej.2014.1624.

26. T. Moro et al., "Effects of Eight Weeks of Time-restricted Feeding (16/8) on Basal Metabolism, Maximal Strength, Body Composition, Inflammation, and Cardiovascular Risk Factors in Resistance-Trained Males," *Journal of Translational Medicine* 14, no. 1 (2016). DOI: 10.1186/s12967-016-1044-0.

27. O. Carlson et al., "Impact of Reduced Meal Frequency Without Caloric Restriction on Glucose Regulation in Healthy, Normal Weight Middle-Aged Men and Women," *Metabolism* 56, no. 12 (December 2007): 1729–734. DOI: 10.1016/j.metabol.2007.07.018.

28. K. S. Stote et al., "A Controlled Trial of Reduced Meal Frequency without Caloric Restriction in Healthy, Normal-Weight, Middle-Aged Adults," *American Journal of Clinical Nutrition* 85, no. 4 (April 2007): 981–88. DOI: 10.1093/ajcn/85.4.981.

29. M. C. Klempel et al., "Intermittent Fasting Combined with Calorie Restriction Is Effective for Weight Loss and Cardio-Protection in Obese Women," *Nutrition Journal* 11, no. 1 (2012). DOI: 10.1186/1475-2891-11-98.

30. T. Moro et al., "Effects of Eight Weeks of Time-restricted Feeding (16/8) on Basal Metabolism, Maximal Strength, Body Composition, Inflammation, and Cardiovascular Risk Factors in Resistance-Trained Males," *Journal of Translational Medicine* 14, no. 1 (2016). DOI: 10.1186/s12967-016-1044-0.

31. G. Tinsley et al., "Time-Restricted Feeding in Young Men Performing Resistance Training: A Randomized Controlled Trial," *European Journal of Sport Science* 17, no. 2 (2016): 200–07. DOI: 10.1080/17461391.2016.1223173.

32. E. C. Westman et al., "The Effect of a Low-Carbohydrate, Ketogenic Diet versus a Low-Glycemic Index Diet on Glycemic Control in Type 2 Diabetes Mellitus," *Nutrition and Metabolism* 5 , no. 36 (December 19, 2008). DOI: 10.1186/1743-7075-5-36.

33. M. Lutski et al., "Insulin Resistance and Future Cognitive Performance and Cognitive Decline in Elderly Patients with Cardiovascular Disease," *Journal of Alzheimer's Disease* 57, no. 2 (2017): 633–43. DOI: 10.3233/jad-161016.

34. C. W. Cheng et al., "Prolonged Fasting Reduces IGF-1/PKA to Promote Hematopoietic-Stem-Cell-Based Regeneration and Reverse Immunosuppression," *Cell Stem Cell* 14, no. 6 (2014): 810–23. DOI: 10.1016/j.stem.2014.04.014.

35. V. D. Longo and P. Fabrizio, "Chronological Aging in Saccharomyces Cerevisiae," *Subcellular Biochemistry* 57 (2012): 101–21. DOI: 10.1007/978-94-007-2561-4_5.

36. W. S. J. Yancy et al., "A Low-Carbohydrate, Ketogenic Diet Versus a Low-Fat Diet to Treat Obesity and Hyperlipidemia: A Randomized, Controlled Trial," *Annals of Internal Medicine* 140, no. 10 (2004): 769–777. DOI: 10.1016/s0084 -3954(07)70252-x.

37. M. V. Chakravarthy and F. W. Booth, "Eating, Exercise, and 'Thrifty' Genotypes: Connecting the Dots toward an Evolutionary Understanding of Modern Chronic Diseases," *Journal of Applied Physiology* 96, no. 1 (2004): 3–10. DOI: 10.1152/japplphysiol.00757.2003.

38. V. D. Longo and M. P. Mattson, "Fasting: Molecular Mechanisms and Clinical Applications," *Cell Metabolism* 19, no. 2 (February 4, 2014): 181–92. DOI: 10.1016/j.cmet.2013.12.008.

39. C-W Cheng, V. Villani, R. Buono, et al., "Fasting-mimicking Diet Promotes Ngn3-driven β-cell Regeneration to Reverse Diabetes," *Cell* 168, no. 5 (2017): 775–788. DOI:10.1016/j.cell.2017.01.040.

40. J. Weisenberger, "Resistant Starch - This Type of Fiber Can Improve Weight Control and Insulin Sensitivity," *Today's Dietitian* 14, no. 9 (September 2012): 22. https://www.todaysdietitian.com/newarchives/090112p22.shtml, accessed 10/20/18.

41. P. M. Smith et al., "The Microbial Metabolites, Short-Chain Fatty Acids, Regulate Colonic Treg Cell Homeostasis," *Science* 341, no. 6145 (August 02, 2013): 569–573. http://science.sciencemag.org/content/341/6145/569, accessed on October 20, 2018.

42. M. T. Streppel et al., "Dietary Fiber and Blood Pressure: A Meta-analysis of Randomized Placebo-Controlled Trials," *Archives of Internal Medicine* 165, no. 2 (January 24, 2005): 150–56. DOI: 10.1001/archinte.165.2.150.

43. WebMD, "Fiber Fights Hypertension?" CBS News, March 04, 2005, https://www.cbsnews.com/news/fiber-fights-hypertension/, accessed 10/20/18.

44. V. Greenwood, Quanta Magazine, "How Bacteria May Help Regulate Blood Pressure," *Scientific American,* December 14, 2017, https://www.scientificamerican.com/article/how-bacteria-may-help-regulate-blood-pressure/, accessed 10/20/18.

45. E. B. Rimm et al., "Vegetable, Fruit, and Cereal Fiber Intake and Risk of Coronary Heart Disease Among Men," *JAMA* 275, no. 6 (1996): 447. DOI: 10.1001/jama.1996.03530300031036.

46. D. F. Birt et al., "Resistant Starch: Promise for Improving Human Health," *Advances in Nutrition* 4, no. 6 (November 2013), https://academic.oup.com/advances/article/4/6/587/4595564, accessed 10/20/18.

47. M. Oaklander, "Eat This Carb and You Won't Gain Weight," *Time* May 06, 2016, http://time.com/4318201/carbohydrates-weight-loss-resistant-starch/, accessed 10/20/18.

48. B. P. Gargari et al., "Is There Any Place for Resistant Starch, as Alimentary Prebiotic, for Patients with Type 2 Diabetes?" *Complementary Therapies in Medicine* 23, no. 6 (2015): 810–15. DOI: 10.1016/j.ctim.2015.09.005.

49. S. S. Dronamraju et al., "Cell Kinetics and Gene Expression Changes in Colorectal Cancer Patients given Resistant Starch: A Randomised Controlled Trial," *Gut* 58, no. 3 (March 2009): 413–20. DOI: 10.1136/gut.2008.162933.

50. R. Marion-Letellier, G. Savoye, and S. Ghosh, "IBD: In Food We Trust," *Journal of Crohns and Colitis* 10, no. 11 (2016): 1351–361. DOI: 10.1093/ecco-jcc/jjw106.

51. American Chemical Society, "New Low-calorie Rice Could Help Cut Rising Obesity Rates," https://www.acs.org/content/acs/en/pressroom/newsreleases/2015/march/new-low-calorie-rice-could-help-cut-rising-obesity-rates.html, accessed 10/20/18.

52. P. Burton and H. J. Lightowler, "The Impact of Freezing and Toasting on the Glycaemic Response of White Bread," *European Journal of Clinical Nutrition* 62, no. 5 (2007): 594–99. DOI: 10.1038/sj.ejcn.1602746.

Chapter 8

1. C. Smith-Spangler et al., "Are Organic Foods Safer or Healthier Than Conventional Alternatives?: A Systematic Review," *Annals of Internal Medicine,* September 4, 2012, http://annals.org/aim/article-abstract/1355685/organic -foods-safer-healthier-than-conventional-alternatives-systematic-review.

2. M. Barański et al., "Higher Antioxidant and Lower Cadmium Concentrations and Lower Incidence of Pesticide Residues in Organically Grown Crops: A Systematic Literature Review and Meta-analyses," *British Journal of Nutrition* 112, no. 05 (2014): 794–811. DOI: 10.1017/s0007114514001366.

3. Centers for Disease Control and Prevention, "Cadmium," March 03, 2011, https://www.atsdr.cdc.gov/substances/toxsubstance.asp?toxid=15.

4. J. P. Reganold et al., "Fruit and Soil Quality of Organic and Conventional Strawberry Agroecosystems," *PLoS One,* https://journals.plos.org/plosone /article?id=10.1371/journal.pone.0012346.

5. M. J. Yousefzadeh et al., "Fisetin Is a Senotherapeutic that Extends Health and Lifespan," *EBioMedicine* 36 (2018): 18–28. DOI: 10.1016/j.ebiom.2018.09.015.

6. D. Srednicka-Tober et al., "Composition Differences between Organic and Conventional Meat: A Systematic Literature Review and Meta-analysis," *British Journal of Nutrition* 115 (2016): 994–1011. https://www.cambridge.org /core/services/aop-cambridge-core/content/view/S0007114515005073.

7. D. Srednicka-Tober et al., "Higher PUFA and N-3 PUFA, Conjugated Linoleic Acid, α-tocopherol and Iron, but Lower Iodine and Selenium Concentrations in Organic Milk: A Systematic Literature Review and Meta- and Redundancy Analyses," *British Journal of Nutrition* 115 (2016): 1043–060. https: //www.cambridge.org/core/services/aop-cambridge-core/content/view /S0007114516000349.

8. C. Long and T. Alterman, "Meet Real Free-Range Eggs - Real Food," *Mother Earth News,* October/November 2007, https://www.motherearthnews.com/real -food/free-range-eggs-zmaz07onzgoe, accessed 10/20/18.

9. Environmental Working Group, "EWG's 2018 Shopper's Guide to Pesticides in Produce," https://www.ewg.org/foodnews/, accessed 10/20/18.

10. A. Fischer et al., "Coenzyme Q Regulates the Expression of Essential Genes of the Pathogen- and Xenobiotic-Associated Defense Pathway in *C. Elegans,*" *Journal of Clinical Biochemistry and Nutrition* 57, no. 3 (2015): 171–77. DOI: 10.3164/jcbn.15-46.

11. B. A. Daisley et al., "Microbiota-Mediated Modulation of Organophosphate Insecticide Toxicity by Species-Dependent Interactions with Lactobacilli in a Drosophila Melanogaster Insect Model," *Applied and Environmental Microbiology* 84, no. 9 (2018). DOI: 10.1128/aem.02820-17.

12. B. V. Deepthi et al., "Lactobacillus Plantarum MYS6 Ameliorates Fumonisin B1- Induced Hepatorenal Damage in Broilers," *Frontiers in Microbiology* 8 (2017). DOI: 10.3389/fmicb.2017.02317.

13. J. Robbers and V. E. Tyler, *Tyler's Herbs of Choice: The Therapeutic Use of Phytomedicinals* (Binghamton, NY: Hawthorne Press, 1999).

14. W. Knoss and F. Stolte, "Assessment Report on *Gentiana Lutea* L., Radix," *European Medicines Agency*, November 12, 2009, https://www.ema.europa.eu/documents/herbal-report/assessment-report-gentiana-lutea-l-radix-first-version_en.pdf.

15. S. W. Seo et al., "Taraxacum Officinale Protects Against Cholecystokinin-Induced Acute Pancreatitis in Rats," *World Journal of Gastroenterology* 11, no. 4 (January 28, 2005): 597–99. DOI: 10.3748/wjg.v11.i4.597.

16. C. M. Park, J. Y. Park, and Y. S. Song, "Luteolin and Chicoric Acid, Two Major Constituents of Dandelion Leaf, Inhibit Nitric Oxide and Lipid Peroxide Formation in Lipopolysaccharide-Stimulated RAW 264.7 Cells," *Preventive Nutrition and Food Science* 15, no. 2 (2010): 92–97. DOI: 10.3746/jfn.2010.15.2.092.

17. Y. J. Koh et al., "Anti-Inflammatory Effect of Taraxacum Officinale Leaves on Lipopolysaccharide-Induced Inflammatory Responses in RAW 264.7 Cells," *Journal of Medicinal Food* 13, no. 4 (2010): 870–78. DOI: 10.1089/jmf.2009.1249.

18. J. F. Cheng et al., "Discovery and Structure-Activity Relationship of Coumarin Derivatives as TNF-alpha Inhibitors," *Bioorganic & Medicinal Chemistry Letters* 14, no. 10 (May 17, 2004): 2411–415. DOI: 10.1016/s0960-894x(04)00355-5.

19. J. Shan et al., "Chlorogenic Acid Inhibits Lipopolysaccharide-induced Cyclooxygenase-2 Expression in RAW264.7 Cells through Suppressing NF-κB and JNK/AP-1 Activation," *International Immunopharmacology* 9, no. 9 (August 2009): 1042–048. DOI: 10.1016/j.intimp.2009.04.011.

20. S. Ammar et al., "Spasmolytic and Anti-Inflammatory Effects of Constituents from Hertia Cheirifolia," *Phytomedicine* 16, no. 12 (December 2009): 1156–161. DOI: 10.1016/j.phymed.2009.03.012.

21. P. Apati et al., "In-vitro Effect of Flavonoids from Solidago Canadensis Extract on Glutathione S-transferase," *Journal of Pharmacy and Pharmacology* 58, no. 2 (February 2006): 251–56. DOI: 10.1211/jpp.58.2.0013.

22. K. M. Ashry et al., "Oxidative Stress and Immunotoxic Effects of Lead and Their Amelioration with Myrrh (Commiphora Molmol) Emulsion," *Food and Chemical Toxicology* 48, no. 1 (January 2010): 236–41. DOI: 10.1016/j.fct.2009.10.006.

23. M. W. Sears, "Chelation: Harnessing and Enhancing Heavy Metal Detoxification—A Review," *Scientific World Journal* 2013 (April 18, 2013): 1–13. DOI: 10.1155/2013/219840.

24. J. Mikler et al., "Successful Treatment of Extreme Acute Lead Intoxication," *Toxicology and Industrial Health* 25, no. 2 (May 20, 2009): 137–40. DOI: 10.1177/0748233709104759.

25. M. D. Aldridge, "Acute Iron Poisoning: What Every Pediatric Intensive Case Unit Nurse Should Know," *Dimensions of Critical Care Nursing* 26, no. 2 (2007): 43–48. DOI: 10.1097/00003465-200703000-00001.

26. B. T. Ly, S. Williams, and R. Clark, "Mercuric Oxide Poisoning Treated with Whole-bowel Irrigation and Chelation Therapy." *Annals of Emergency Medicine* 39, no. 3 (March 2002): 312–15. DOI: 10.1067/mem.2002.119508.

27. R. Kumar and N. V. Majeti, "A Review of Chitin and Chitosan Applications," *Reactive and Functional Polymers* 46, no. 1 (November 2000): 1–27. https://www.sciencedirect.com/science/article/abs/pii/S1381514800000389#!.

28. E. Guibal, "Interactions of Metal Ions with Chitosan-based Sorbents: A Review," *Separation and Purification Technology* 38, no. 1 (July 15, 2004): 43–74. DOI: 10.1016/j.seppur.2003.10.004.

29. A. J. Varma, S. V. Deshpande, and J. F. Kennedy, "Metal Complexation by Chitosan and Its Derivatives: A Review," *Carbohydrate Polymers* 55, no. 1 (January 1, 2004): 77–93. DOI: 10.1016/j.carbpol.2003.08.005.

30. L. Zhang, Y. Zeng, and Z. Cheng, "Removal of Heavy Metal Ions Using Chitosan and Modified Chitosan: A Review," *Journal of Molecular Liquids* 214 (February 2016): 175–91. https://www.sciencedirect.com/science/article/pii/S0167732215308801.

31. J. Wang and C. Chen, "Chitosan-Based Biosorbents: Modification and Application for Biosorption of Heavy Metals and Radionuclides," *Bioresource Technology* 160 (May 2014): 129–41. DOI: 10.1016/j.biortech.2013.12.110.

32. T. Fang et al., "Modified Citrus Pectin Inhibited Bladder Tumor Growth through Downregulation of Galectin-3," *Acta Pharmacologica Sinica* (May 16, 2018). DOI: 10.1038/s41401-018-0004-z.

33. Z. Y. Zhao et al., "The Role of Modified Citrus Pectin as an Effective Chelator of Lead in Children Hospitalized with Toxic Lead Levels," *Alternative Therapies in Health and Medicine* 14, no. 4 (July/August 2008): 34–38. https://www.ncbi.nlm.nih.gov/pubmed/18616067.

34. I. Eliaz, E. Weil, and B. Wilk, "Integrative Medicine and the Role of Modified Citrus Pectin/Alginates in Heavy MetIntegrative Medicine and the Role of Modified Citrus Pectin/Alginates in Heavy Metal Chelation and Detoxification – Five Case Reports," *Complementary Medicine Research* 14, no. 6 (December 2007): 358–64. DOI: 10.1159/000109829.

35. T. Uchikawa et al., "Chlorella Suppresses Methylmercury Transfer to the Fetus in Pregnant Mice," *Journal of Toxicological Sciences* 36, no. 5 (October 2011): 675–80. DOI: 10.2131/jts.36.675.

36. J. Mercola and D. Klinghardt, "Mercury Toxicity and Systemic Elimination Agents," *Journal of Nutritional & Environmental Medicine* 11, no. 1 (2001): 53–62. DOI: 10.1080/13590840020030267.

37. O. R. Ajuwon, O. O. Oguntibeju, and J. Lucasta Marnewick, "Amelioration of Lipopolysaccharide-Induced Liver Injury by Aqueous Rooibos (Aspalathus Linearis) Extract via Inhibition of Pro-Inflammatory Cytokines and Oxidative Stress," *BMC Complementary and Alternative Medicine* 14, no. 1 (October 13, 2014). DOI: 10.1186/1472-6882-14-392.

38. Q. Liu et al., "Effects of Dandelion Extract on the Proliferation of Rat Skeletal Muscle Cells and the Inhibition of a Lipopolysaccharide-Induced Inflammatory Reaction," *Chinese Medical Journal* 131, no. 14 (July 20, 2018): 1724–731. DOI: 10.4103/0366-6999.235878.

39. M. W. Ebada, "Essential Oils of Green Cumin and Chamomile Partially Protect against Acute Acetaminophen Hepatotoxicity in Rats," *Anais Da Academia Brasileira De Ciências* 90, no. 2 Suppl 1 (June 25, 2018): 2347–358. DOI: 10.1590/0001-3765201820170825.

40. M. Ogata et al., "Supplemental Psyllium Fibre Regulates the Intestinal Barrier and Inflammation in Normal and Colitic Mice," *British Journal of Nutrition* 118, no. 09 (November 2017): 661–72. DOI: 10.1017/s0007114517002586.

Chapter 9

1. S. L. McDonnell et al., "Serum 25-Hydroxyvitamin D Concentrations ≥40 Ng/ml Are Associated with 65% Lower Cancer Risk: Pooled Analysis of Randomized Trial and Prospective Cohort Study," *PLoS One* 11, no. 4 (2016). https://www .ncbi.nlm.nih.gov/pmc/articles/PMC4822815/, accessed 10/20/2018.

2. M. Garlapow, "Higher Vitamin D Levels Lower Risk of Cancer in Women," OncologyNurseAdvisor, April 22, 2016, http://www.oncologynurseadvisor .com/colorectal-cancer/vitamin-d-and-cancer-higher-levels-lower-risk-in- women/article/491569/, accessed 10/20/2018.

3. University of California, San Diego, "Greater Levels of Vitamin D Associated with Decreasing Risk of Breast Cancer," ScienceDaily, June 15, 2018, https: //www.sciencedaily.com/releases/2018/06/180615154523.htm, accessed 10/20/2018.

4. "Game Changer of the Year: Carole Baggerly," Mercola.com, https://articles .mercola.com/sites/articles/archive/2018/08/07/game-changer-of-the-year -carole-baggerly.aspx, accessed 10/20/2018.

5. "Lower Disease Incidence with Vitamin D levels 40-60 ng/ml," GrassrootsHealth, https://grassrootshealth.net/project/general-health/, accessed 10/20/2018.

6. C. F. Garland et al., "Vitamin D Supplement Doses and Serum 25-hydroxyvitamin D in the Range Associated with Cancer Prevention," *Anticancer Research* 31, no. 2 (February 2011): 607–11, https://www.ncbi.nlm. nih.gov/pubmed/21378345.

7. "Foods Highest in Vitamin D," SELF Nutrition Data, http://nutritiondata.self .com/foods-000102000000000000000.html, accessed 10/20/18.

8. J. J. DiNicolantonio, J. H. O'Keefe, and W. Wilson, "Subclinical Magnesium Deficiency: A Principal Driver of Cardiovascular Disease and a Public Health Crisis," *Open Heart* 5, no. 1 (2018). DOI: 10.1136/openhrt-2017-000668corr1.

9. Y. H. Ko et al., "Chemical Mechanism of ATP Synthase," *Journal of Biological Chemistry* 274, no. 41 (1999): 28853–8856. DOI: 10.1074/jbc.274.41.28853.

10. A. S. Mildvan, "Role of Magnesium and Other Divalent Cations in ATP- Utilizing Enzymes." *Magnesium* 6, no. 1 (1987): 28–33. https://www.ncbi .nlm.nih.gov/pubmed/3029516.

11. J. Wang et al., "Dietary Magnesium Intake Improves Insulin Resistance among Non-Diabetic Individuals with Metabolic Syndrome Participating in a Dietary Trial," *Nutrients* 5, no. 10 (2013): 3910–919. DOI: 10.3390/nu5103910.

12. K. Maeshima et al., "A Transient Rise in Free Mg^{2+} Ions Released from ATP- Mg Hydrolysis Contributes to Mitotic Chromosome Condensation," *Current Biology* 28, no. 3 (2018). DOI: 10.1016/j.cub.2017.12.035.

13. A. A. Zheltova et al., "Magnesium Deficiency and Oxidative Stress: An Update," *BioMedicine* 6, no. 4 (2016). DOI: 10.7603/s40681-016-0020-6.

14. USDA National Nutrient Database for Standard Reference Release 28, November 10, 2015, https://ods.od.nih.gov/pubs/usdandb/Magnesium-Content.pdf.

15. S. Johnson, "The Multifaceted and Widespread Pathology of Magnesium Deficiency," *Medical Hypotheses* 56, no. 2 (2001): 163–70. DOI: 10.1054 /mehy.2000.1133.

16. NIH Office of Dietary Supplements, "Magnesium," https://ods.od.nih.gov /factsheets/Magnesium-HealthProfessional/.

17. J. J. DiNicolantonio, J. H. O'Keefe, and W. Wilson, "Subclinical Magnesium Deficiency: A Principal Driver of Cardiovascular Disease and a Public Health Crisis," *Open Heart* 5, no. 1 (2018). DOI: 10.1136/openhrt-2017-000668corr1.

18. A. M. Uwitonze and M. S. Razzaque, "Role of Magnesium in Vitamin D Activation and Function," *Journal of the American Osteopathic Association* 118, no. 3 (2018): 181. DOI: 10.7556/jaoa.2018.037.

19. American Osteopathic Association, "Researchers Find Low Magnesium Levels Make Vitamin D Ineffective," EurekAlert! https://www.eurekalert.org/pub_ releases/2018-02/aoa-rfl022318.php.

20. Ibid.

21. X. Deng et al., "Magnesium, Vitamin D Status and Mortality: Results from US National Health and Nutrition Examination Survey (NHANES) 2001 to 2006 and NHANES III," *BMC Medicine* 11, no. 1 (2013). DOI: 10.1186/1741-7015-11 -187.

22. W. S. Harris et al., "Erythrocyte Long-Chain Omega-3 Fatty Acid Levels Are Inversely Associated with Mortality and with Incident Cardiovascular Disease: The Framingham Heart Study," *Journal of Clinical Lipidology* 12, no. 3 (2018). DOI: 10.1016/j.jacl.2018.02.010.

23. S. M. Ulven et al., "Metabolic Effects of Krill Oil Are Essentially Similar to Those of Fish Oil but at Lower Dose of EPA and DHA, in Healthy Volunteers," *Lipids* 46, no. 1 (2010): 37–46. DOI: 10.1007/s11745-010-3490-4.

24. Mayo Clinic, "Prediabetes," August 02, 2017, https://www.mayoclinic.org /diseases-conditions/prediabetes/symptoms-causes/syc-20355278, accessed 10/20/18.

25. "#LCHF The Genius of Dr. Joseph R. Kraft - Exposing the True Extent of #Diabetes," The Fat Emperor, http://www.thefatemperor.com/blog/2015/5/10 /lchf-the-genius-of-dr-joseph-r-kraft-exposing-the-true-extent-of-diabetes, accessed 10/20/18.

26. F. S. Facchini, "Near-Iron Deficiency-Induced Remission of Gouty Arthritis," *Rheumatology* 42, no. 12 (2003): 1550–555. DOI: 10.1093/rheumatology /keg402.

27. Iron Disorders Institute, http://www.irondisorders.org/, accessed 10/20/18.

28. J. Daru et al., "Serum Ferritin Thresholds for the Diagnosis of Iron Deficiency in Pregnancy: A Systematic Review," *Transfusion Medicine* 27, no. 3 (2017): 167–74. DOI: 10.1111/tme.12408.

29. G. Koenig and S. Seneff, "Gamma-Glutamyltransferase: A Predictive Biomarker of Cellular Antioxidant Inadequacy and Disease Risk," *Disease Markers* 2015 (2015): 1–18. DOI: 10.1155/2015/818570.

30. "What Is a Hs-CRP Test, and Do You Need One?" MedBroadcast.com, https://www.medbroadcast.com/channel/cholesterol/testing-testing/what-is-a-hs-crp-test-and-do-you-need-one, accessed 10/20/18.

31. J. L. Funk et al., "Efficacy and Mechanism of Action of Turmeric Supplements in the Treatment of Experimental Arthritis," *Arthritis & Rheumatism* 54, no. 11 (2006): 3452–464. DOI: 10.1002/art.22180.

32. J. Younger, L. Parkitny, and D. McLain, "The Use of Low-Dose Naltrexone (LDN) as a Novel Anti-Inflammatory Treatment for Chronic Pain," *Clinical Rheumatology* 33, no. 4 (2014): 451–59. DOI: 10.1007/s10067-014-2517-2.

33. "CLIA Program and HIPAA Privacy Rule; Patients' Access to Test Reports," *Federal Register* February 6, 2014, https://www.federalregister.gov/documents/2014/02/06/2014-02280/clia-program-and-hipaa-privacy-rule-patients-access-to-test-reports, accessed 10/20/18.

INDEX

long-term ketosis and, 101–102

lowering intake, and becoming metabolically flexible, 34–35, 91–92

as primary fuel, problem with, xii

threshold level, determining, 118

Charcoal, activated, as binder, 136–137

characteristics and impacts of, 51–54

exposure to resulting from fasting, 73

glyphosate, 6–7, 53–54, 70, 106. *See also* Herbicides and pesticides

polychlorinated biphenyls (PCBs), 71, 72, 75

POPs, 70–72, 73, 74–75

removing. *See* Detoxification

synthetic fertilizers, 5–6

water fasting precaution, 51–52

Chemotherapy, water fasting and, 65

Chitosan, as binder, 137

Chlorella, as binder, 137–138

Cholesterol, xi, 15, 90, 151, 152–153

Christianity, fasting and, 21–22

The Circadian Code (Panda), 12

app for tracking, 59

gut health and, 42–43

timing of food intake and, 12–16, 42, 59

Citrus pectin, modified, 137

Coconut and MCT oil, 131–133

Coffee and additives, for KetoFast days, 139, 140

The Complete Guide to Fasting (Fung), 34, 51

Contraindications for KetoFasting, 66–67

Cronometer, 99–100, 120–123, 130–131, 134, 138

Cyclical ketogenic diet, 89–108. *See also* Feasting/feast days

about: overview and summary, 89–91, 108

benefits of nutritional ketosis, 97–98

continuous keto diet vs., xiii

fats to eat and not eat, 100–101

following on non-fasting days, 77

glucose vs. ketones and, 95–96

how to eat for ketosis, 99–100

importance of varying/taking breaks from, 90–91

metabolic flexibility importance, 92–95. *See also* Metabolic flexibility

switching to. *See* Cyclical ketogenic diet, making switch to

switching to burning for fuel. *See also* Cyclical ketogenic diet, making switch to

tracking nutrient intake on cronometer, 99–100, 120–123, 130–131, 134, 138

TRE study and, 89–90

value of switching to burning fat, 91

variety importance and, 102–103

Cyclical ketogenic diet, making switch to, 115–128

about: overview of, 115–116

body fat percentage determination and guidelines, 123–126

ketone monitoring devices and accessories, 116–117

monitoring long-term progress, 118

safest sugar alternatives for, 126–128

tracking food intake on cronometer, 120–123

when to monitor ketones, 117–118

D

Dandelion, for detox, 135–136

Dandelion root tea, 139

Dark side of fasting. *See* Chemical toxins; Toxins

Detoxification

active vs passive sweating and, 78–79

fasting benefits, 41–42

of heavy metals, 72–73

how body detoxes harmful substances, 75–79

with KetoFasting, xv, xvi

lipolysis and, xvi, 35, 41, 57, 69, 76

phases (stages) of, 76–78

resource to help, xvii

sauna therapy for. *See* Saunas

side effects, 57

supplements to support, 133–136, 145

sweating to remove toxins from body, 77, 78–79. *See also* Sweating

teas for, 139

DEXA scan, 125–126

Diabetes. *See also* Insulin resistance

fasting benefits, 44, 92, 103, 148–149

fasting blood insulin test, 148–149

foolish medical strategy for, 34

ketogenic diet and, 97

Diabetes Epidemic & You (Kraft), 4, 34

Dioxins and dioxin-like chemicals, 52

Disease (chronic)

about: overview and summary, 1–3, 16–17

conventional medical approach, 1–2

dietary changes leading to, 3–5

diseases considered "chronic," 2

electromagnetic fields (EMFs) and, 7–9

food additives and, 6

healthcare cost impact, 2

inflammation and, 10–12

iron excess and, 9

microbiome changes and, 10

pesticides and, 6–7. *See also* Glyphosate; Herbicides and pesticides

POPs and, 70–71. *See also* Persistent organic pollutants (POPs)

prevalence of, 1–2

reversing through fasting, 3

synthetic fertilizers and, 6

as top causes of death, 2

Dual-energy X-ray absorptiometry (DEXA) scan, 125–126

E

Electromagnetic fields (EMFs), 7–9

Esser, William, N.D., D.C., 29

The Every-Other-Day Diet (Varady), 58

Evolution, fasting and, 19–20

Exercise, stimulating autophagy with, 37

F

Fasting. *See also* Intermittent fasting; KetoFasting

basic categories of, 49–51

best first step toward, 15

dark side of. *See* Chemical toxins; Toxins

getting to homeostasis, 3

history of. *See* History of fasting

importance of, xiv

safety considerations, 63–69. *See also* Chemical toxins; Toxins

side effects of, 64–65

stem cells running on, 40–41

timing of your food and, xiv

types of, 49–61

Fasting: An Exceptional Human Experience (Fredricks), 20

Fat

benefits of burning for fuel, xii

H

I

P

Panda, Dr. Satchin, 12, 14–15, 59

Paracelsus, on fasting, 27

Partial fasting, about, 50. *See also* KetoFasting

Passive vs active sweating, 78–79

PBDEs, 71

PCBs. *See* Polychlorinated biphenyls

Peak Fasting, 35, 49, 55–56

Percent of body fat, determining, 123–126

Persistent organic pollutants (POPs), 70–72, 73, 74–75

Pesticides. *See* Herbicides and pesticides

Phases of detoxification, 76–78

Phosphatidylcholine, 134, 135

Photo, for body fat approximation, 124

Plato, on fasting, 27

Polychlorinated biphenyls (PCBs), 71, 72, 75

Polycyclic aromatic hydrocarbons, 52

POPs. *See* Persistent organic pollutants

Pregnancy, KetoFasting and, 66

Probiotics, 134

Protein

calculating grams needed, 123

chlorella algae for, 137–138

cyclical ketogenesis and, xiii

HS-CRP test, 150–151

for ketosis, 99, 104, 106–107, 108

liver, test for C-reactive protein, 150–151

more on feast days, 106–107

stimulating autophagy with AMPK, 37–38

tracking intake of, 120

Psyllium, 133, 140–141

R

Ramayana, fasting and, 26

Reactive oxygen species (ROS), 10, 11, 13, 15, 44, 70, 96, 97

Recipes, choosing, 130–131

Religious fasting, 21–25

Resources, 155–156

Rooibos tea, 139

Rumi, on fasting, 23

S

Safety of fasting, 63–69

Sauna Therapy for Detoxification and Healing (Wilson), 86

Saunas, 79–86

about: overview of, 79

activating bodily healing, 80–81

active vs passive sweating and, 78–79

buying/building your own, 83–84

cold plunge after, 84–85

far-IR misrepresentations, 81–82

incandescent near-IR heating benefits, 82

near-IR vs. far-IR, 79–82

post-sauna rinse, 84–85

reference book on using, 86

safety guidelines, 85–86

showering after, 84

therapeutic dosing, 83

Scale, digital food, 119–120

Scale, digital with body fat readings, 125

Serum ferritin test and effects, 149–150

Shelton, Herbert M., D.C., N.D., 29

SIBO (small intestinal bowel overgrowth), 110, 111

Side effects of fasting, 64–65

Skin calipers, for body fat percentage, 124–125

Sleep

chamomile tea before, 139

downsides of eating close to, 5, 15

fasting improving, 28

U

Ubiquinol (CoQ10), 133

Uric acid (high), KetoFasting and, 67

V

Varady, Krista, 58

Variety, importance of, 102–103

Vitamin D level, 144–145

W

Water fasting

about, 50–51

chemotherapy and, 65

compliance problem, xvi

effectiveness of, 65

harmful chemical toxins impacting, 51–54

KetoFasting vs., xvi–xvii, 77

largest North American clinic, 29, 30

precautions/safety considerations, 51–54, 63–64

regaining fat-burning ability after, 35–36

Water, for KetoFast days, 138, 139

Weight, contraindication for fasting, 66, 68

Weight loss

adaptive thermogenesis and, 74

cyclical ketogenic diet and, 90, 98

fasting and, 43–44, 53, 58, 73

increased POPs in blood and, 74, 75

timing of food intake, circadian rhythms and, 12, 14–15

toxic exposure from, 73

why people don't maintain, 74

Why We Sleep (Walker), 14

X

X-ray (DEXA scan), 125–126

ACKNOWLEDGMENTS

My deepest appreciation for the two primary editors who helped create this book. Kate Hanley is a brilliant, kind, and talented writer who skillfully helped craft my recommendations into text.

Janet Selvig was the other primary editor. Janet is my sister, and I love her dearly. She started my medical practice with me in 1985, and was my first employee. She continues to work as the chief editor of our website. I can always count on her to give me honest and highly insightful edits. I don't know what I would do without her.

Alan Goldhamer, D.C., is the medical director of the True North Clinic in California, the largest water fasting clinic in North America. He provided much of the foundational research on the history of fasting in this book.

ABOUT THE AUTHOR

Dr. Joseph Mercola is a physician and *New York Times* best-selling author. He was voted the Ultimate Wellness Game Changer by the Huffington Post and has been featured in several national media outlets, including *Time* magazine, the *Los Angeles Times*, CNN, Fox News, ABC News, *TODAY*, and *The Dr. Oz Show*. His mission is to transform the traditional medical paradigm in the United States into one in which the root cause of disease is treated, rather than the symptoms. In addition, he aims to expose corporate and government fraud and mass media hype that often sends people down an unhealthy path.

Hay House Titles of Related Interest

YOU CAN HEAL YOUR LIFE,
the movie, starring Louise Hay & Friends
(available as a 1-DVD program, an expanded 2-DVD set,
and an online streaming video)
Learn more at www.hayhouse.com/louise-movie

THE SHIFT, the movie,
starring Dr. Wayne W. Dyer
(available as a 1-DVD program, an expanded 2-DVD set,
and an online streaming video)
Learn more at www.hayhouse.com/the-shift-movie

***

THE ALLERGY SOLUTION: Unlock the Surprising Hidden Truth about Why You are Sick and How to Get Well, by Leo Galland, M.D.

COMPLETE KETO: A Guide to Transforming Your Body and Your Mind for Life, by Drew Manning

FEEDING YOU LIES: How to Unravel the Food Industry's Playbook and Reclaim Your Health, by Vani Hari

YOUNG AND SLIM FOR LIFE: 10 Essential Steps to Achieve Total Vitality and Kick-Start Weight Loss That Lasts, by Dr. Frank Lipman

All of the above are available at your local bookstore,
or may be ordered by contacting Hay House (see next page).

***

We hope you enjoyed this Hay House book. If you'd like to receive our online catalog featuring additional information on Hay House books and products, or if you'd like to find out more about the Hay Foundation, please contact:

Hay House, Inc., P.O. Box 5100, Carlsbad, CA 92018-5100
(760) 431-7695 or (800) 654-5126
(760) 431-6948 (fax) or (800) 650-5115 (fax)
www.hayhouse.com® • www.hayfoundation.org

———

Published in Australia by: Hay House Australia Pty. Ltd.,
18/36 Ralph St., Alexandria NSW 2015
Phone: 612-9669-4299 • *Fax:* 612-9669-4144
www.hayhouse.com.au

Published in the United Kingdom by: Hay House UK, Ltd.,
The Sixth Floor, Watson House, 54 Baker Street, London W1U 7BU
Phone: +44 (0)20 3927 7290 • *Fax:* +44 (0)20 3927 7291
www.hayhouse.co.uk

Published in India by: Hay House Publishers India,
Muskaan Complex, Plot No. 3, B-2, Vasant Kunj, New Delhi 110 070
Phone: 91-11-4176-1620 • *Fax:* 91-11-4176-1630
www.hayhouse.co.in

———

Access New Knowledge.
Anytime. Anywhere.

Learn and evolve at your own pace
with the world's leading experts.

www.hayhouseU.com

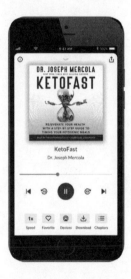